Health Improvement Library
Law House
Airdrie Road
Carluke
M18 5ER

Key Concepts in
Public Health

FRANCES WILSON AND
MZWANDILE MABHALA

Key Concepts in
Public Health

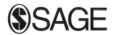

Los Angeles • London • New Delhi • Singapore • Washington DC

SAGE Publications Ltd
1 Oliver's Yard
55 City Road
London EC1Y 1SP

SAGE Publications Inc.
2455 Teller Road
Thousand Oaks, California 91320

SAGE Publications India Pvt Ltd
B 1/I 1 Mohan Cooperative Industrial Area
Mathura Road, New Delhi 110 044

SAGE Publications Asia-Pacific Pte Ltd
33 Pekin Street #02-01
Far East Square
Singapore 048763

Library of Congress Control Number: 2008926948

British Library Cataloguing in Publication data

A catalogue record for this book is available from the
British Library

ISBN 978-1-4129-4879-1
ISBN 978-1-4129-4880-7 (pbk)

Typeset by C&M Digitals (P) Ltd, Chennai, India
Printed in Great Britain by The Cromwell Press Ltd, Trowbridge, Wiltshire
Printed on paper from sustainable resources

contents

contents

v

key concepts in
public health

vi

contents

editors and contributors

Editors

Mzwandile (Andi) Mabhala FRIPH, M.Sc.(PH), B.Sc. (Hons) PG Cert. Ed. is Senior Lecturer in Public Health and Epidemiology, Faculty of Health and Social Care, University of Chester and Fellow of the Royal Institute of Public Health.

Frances Wilson M.Sc., B.Sc., PG Dip Ed., RGN, RM, SCPHN is Senior Lecturer and Programme Leader, M.Sc. Health Improvement and Wellbeing and Pathway Leader, Specialist Community Public Health Nursing (Health Visiting), Faculty of Health and Social Care, University of Chester.

Authors

Hamed A. Adetunji B.Sc., Dip. (Epid)., M.Sc. (Epid)., MPH, Ph.D., PGCHE, FRIPH is Course Leader, M.Sc. Public Health, Oxford Brookes University.

Fiona Adshead B.Sc., MB BS, FRCP, M.Sc., FFPH is Deputy Chief Medical Officer in the Department of Health for England and the Chief Government Adviser on Health Inequalities.

Edward Andersson MA, MSc. is Project Manager at Involve, London.

Moyra Baldwin B.Sc. (Hons), M.MedSci. (Clinical Nursing), RN (Adult), RCNT, RT, Dip. N. (London), Cert. Ed, Dip. Adv. Nursing Studies, JBCNS 100, ENB 931 is Senior Lecturer and Programme Leader of the Post Graduate Certificate in Health and Social Care Commissioning, Faculty of Health and Social Care, University of Chester.

Tina Barrows RGN. Dip. RHV. B.Sc. (Hons) Community Health. Adult Cert. Ed. is Senior Lecturer in the Faculty of Health and Social Care at the University of Chester and Specialist Community Public Health Nurse (Health Visiting), Warrington (NHS) Community Services Unit.

Sara Bell RNLD, BA (Hons), Specialist Practitioner is Senior Lecturer in Learning Disability Nursing and Programme Leader, Specialist Practitioner Qualification in Community Learning Disability Nursing, Faculty of Health and Social Care, University of Chester.

Clive Blair-Stevens B.Sc., CQSW, ASW is co-founder of the National Social Marketing Centre based in London, and its Director of Strategy and Operations.

Ann Bryan M.Sc., Cert. Ed., ADM, RGN, RM, HV, RMT is Head of Community and Child Health, Faculty of Health and Social Care, University of Chester.

Pat Clarke B.Sc. (Hons) Health Studies, RGN, RM, RHV is health visitor and professional development nurse, Wirral PCT.

Nicola Close MA (Oxon), MA (Bham), FRIPH, FRSS, MIHM is Chief Executive, Association of Directors of Public Health, Fellow of the Royal Institute of Public Health and of the Royal Statistical Society and Member of the Institute of Healthcare Management.

Irene Cooke RGN, RM, MPH, DN, B.Sc. (Hons), PGCHE, CPNP is Senior Lecturer in Public Health and Community Nursing, Programme Lead for the B.Sc./PG Dip./M.Sc. Specialist Practitioner in Community Nursing Programmes, Faculty of Health and Social Care, University of Chester.

David Coyle RN, M.Ed Cert. Ed. is Senior Lecturer in Mental Health, Faculty of Health and Social Care, University of Chester.

Diane Crone B.Sc. (Hons), Ph.D. is Reader in Exercise Science, Faculty of Sport, Health and Social Care, University of Gloucestershire and is a BASES accredited exercise scientist (support and research).

Pat Deeny RN, B.Sc. (Hons) Nursing, Adv. Dip. Ed., RNT is Senior Lecturer in the School of Nursing, University of Ulster.

Walid El Ansari MBBCH, Dip. (P. Ed.), DTM&H, M.Sc. (PHM), PG Cert. (HE), Ph.D. (Wales), Ph.D. (Oxford Brookes), FRIPH is Professor and Head of Public Health, Faculty of Sport, Health and Social Care, University of Gloucestershire.

Basma Ellahi RPHNutr., MIFST, Ph.D, M.Sc., B.Sc., Pg Cert is Head of Department of Biological Sciences, University of Chester.

Michelle Falconer MPH, BN (Hons), RGN, DN Cert. is Immunisation Co-ordinator for Halton & St Helens PCT.

Jeff French Ph.D., MBA, M.Sc., Dip. HE, BA, Cert. Ed. is Director of the National Social Marketing Centre and a Fellow at Kings College, London.

Kim Greening MA, BSc.(Hons), Dip. Mgmt, PGCE, RN, HV Dip. is Deputy Head of Department – Practice Learning, Development and Allied Healthcare, Faculty of Health & Social Care, University of Chester.

Jan Hardy RGN, RM, SPCHN, B.Sc. Professional Practice (Public Health), PGDE is Senior Lecturer, Faculty of Health and Social Care, University of Chester.

Scott Harrison RN, RHV, B.Sc. (Hons), MA is Public Health Nursing Supervisor at Fraser Health Authority, Vancouver, Canada.

Elaine Hogard Ph.D. MA, M.Sc., BA (Hons) is Professor of Evaluation Research in the Social and Health Evaluation Unit, Faculty of Education and Children's Services, University of Chester.

Graham Holroyd M.Sc., BA (Hons), Dip. ASCE (Dist.), MIHEP, Fellow Higher Education Academy is Senior Lecturer and Course Leader in the School of Health and Postgraduate Medicine at the University of Central Lancashire, an Associate Lecturer, School of Health and Social Care, Open University and Chair of the European Men's Health Research Network.

John Horley RN (Child) Dip. HE (nursing) M.Sc. (APNP) is Lecturer in Community and Child Health, Faculty of Health and Social Care, University of Chester.

Mike Horah BA (Hons) is career civil servant in the Department of Health and acting Policy Adviser to the National Social Marketing Centre, National Consumer Council.

Richard Jarvis MBBS, B.Sc., MPH, PG Dip.Sci. (Environmental Protection) FFPH is Consultant in Health Protection, Cheshire and Merseyside Health Protection Unit.

Peete Lesiamo PG Cert., BA HRM, B.Ed. Education in Development, BA ED is a Public Health Practitioner, Pholokoeo, South Africa.

Gail Louw Ph.D, BA, MA, M.Sc. is Principal Lecturer and Public Health Programme Leader, Institute of Postgraduate Medicine, Brighton and Sussex Medical School.

Andy Lovell Ph.D., BA (Hons), Cert. Ed., RNLD is Reader in Learning Disabilities, Faculty of Health and Social Care, University of Chester

Judith Lydon RN, RHV, SN, B.Sc. (Hons), P.G Cert. is Community Matron for Vulnerable Adults, Warrington PCT.

Jean Mannix M.Ed. Professional Education, B.Sc. (Hons), RGN, SCPHN, HV, Nurse Prescriber is Deputy Head of the Community and Child Health Department and Programme Leader M.Sc./PGD/B.Sc. (Hons) Specialist Community Public Health Nursing programme, Faculty of Health and Social Care, University of Chester.

Elizabeth Mason-Whitehead Ph.D., BA (Hons), HV, PGDE, ONC, SRN, SCM is Reader in Community Studies, Faculty of Health and Social Care, University of Chester.

Alan Massey M.Sc. in Public Health and Health Promotion; B.Sc. (Hons), SCPHN (Occupational Health) is Senior Lecturer in the Faculty of Health and Social Care, University of Chester.

Jill McCarthy M.Sc., B.Ed. (Hons), RGN, DN, RNT is Senior Lecturer, and Programme Leader, M.Sc. in Professional Practice, Faculty of Health and Social Care, University of Chester.

Rowena Merritt D.Phil. is Practitioners Development Programme Manager, National Social Marketing Centre.

Hayley Mills B.Sc. (Hons), M.Sc. is Ph.D. candidate, Faculty of Sport, Health and Social Care, University of Gloucestershire.

Sue Phillips RGN, RHV, BA (Hons) Nursing Education, M.Sc. Primary Healthcare is Senior Lecturer and AP(E)L/Work Based Learning Co-ordinator, Faculty of Health and Social Care, University of Chester.

Nicholas Fulton Phin MB, CLB, LLM, FFPHM is Consultant Epidemiologist, Respiratory Virus Infection (influenza and SARS), Health Protection Agency, Centre for Infections, London.

Dianne Phipps MA, PGCE, RNMH is Deputy Head of Department – Mental Health and Learning Disabilities, Faculty of Health and Social Care, University of Chester.

Gabrielle Rabie RMN, SRN, SCPHN, MPH is Senior Lecturer, Programme Lead for Youth Matters, Pathway Lead, School of Nursing, Faculty of Health and Social Care, University of Chester.

Pat Rose RN, SCPHN (HV), M.Sc., B.Sc., Dip.N., Cert. Ed. is Senior Lecturer, Faculty of Health and Social Care, University of Chester.

Soumen Sengupta B.Sc. (Hons), M.Sc. is Head of Planning and Health Improvement, NHS Greater Glasgow and Clyde, West Dunbartonshire Community Health Partnership.

Alex G. Stewart MB, Ch.B., MPH, MFPHMI, MFPH, DRCOG, DTM&H, FHEA is Consultant in Health Protection, Cheshire & Merseyside Health Protection Unit.

Janine Talley Ph.D., MA, B.Sc., PGCE is Staff Tutor, Faculty of Health and Social Care, Open University working in health and management.

Mike Thomas Ph.D., MA (Law), B. Nurs., RMN, RNT, Cert. Ed., MILT is Professor of Eating Disorders and Dean, Faculty of Health and Social Care, University of Chester.

Allison Thorpe M.Sc. (PH), MRIPH, B.Sc. (Hons) is Policy Manager, National Social Marketing Centre.

Rachel A. Wells MPH, M.Sc. is Consultant in Public Health, member of the Voluntary Register for Public Health, Fellow of the Faculty of Public Health and member of the UKPHA.

acknowledgements

The editors would like to thank their colleagues at University of Chester for their support and encouragement.

Frances would like to thank her husband Michael for his unstinting support.

Andi would like to thank Melanie for her fortitude.

Introduction

Significant changes occurring in the organisation and practice of public health demand a fresh look at some of the established public health concepts, as well as a consideration of new and emerging themes.

Assuming no previous experience of public health and minimal knowledge of public health concepts, theories, principles and domains, this is the ideal guide for those new to the public health field. It is essential reading for those involved in public health practice. It will also appeal to a wider audience of professionals, lay people and students who are interested in public and community health.

Key Concepts can support programmes of study, or readers may use the book as a reference point, for supplementary reading or to provide an introduction to a specific concept. Public health lecturers, particularly undergraduate lecturers, can use this book to inform their teaching. Examples of appropriate programmes may include undergraduate degrees in community and specialist practice community nursing and public health where the emphasis is on application of theory to practice, as well as more generic foundation degrees. This book will meet a need in this new market, providing a succinct introduction to theoretical concepts and practical applications that students can then build on to meet their specific requirements.

The book aims:

- To introduce undergraduate students to the key concepts of public health.
- To reacquaint public health practitioners and the wider public health workforce with the key concepts of public health.
- To be used as a source book and educational tool for lecturers involved in teaching public health.

The concepts are organised into sections based on the knowledge that students, public health practitioners and the wider public health workforce need to support practice; practical applications of the concepts; and broader concepts affecting specific populations.

The concepts will be grouped into the following sections:

- **Theoretical Concepts** – the building blocks for public health practice. These will consist of common subject areas for definition and discussion, explaining how and why these concepts are necessary for public health practice.
- **Practical Concepts** – for application/implementation and evaluation of public health practice. These will have a practical focus with case history examples to illustrate application of the concept.
- **Populations and Public Health Practice** – This section will look at public health of populations, focusing on their specific needs using settings approaches where relevant.

Public health is often perceived as theoretical with no clear application of theory to practice; this book aims to explicitly demonstrate this application of theory through the use of case studies and application to practice examples.

Frances Wilson and Andi Mabhala

key concepts
in public health

2

Part I
Theoretical Concepts

1 The Historical Development of Public Health

Nicholas Fulton Phin

DEFINITION

The association between human disease and the growth of centres of population has long been observed and the concept of action at a community or population level to influence health is not new; the Romans incorporated aqueducts and sewage systems into the design of their cities. However, for this chapter, the historical focus will be on the emergence of the modern public health movement from the 1830s onward.

KEY POINTS

- Early public health work focused on the prevention of infectious diseases; the focus is now on other determinants of health.
- Many of the greatest successes of public health were achieved when the public health department was within and able to influence local government.
- Is the health service, with its emphasis on treatment and care, the right base for a modern public health service?

DISCUSSION

The Industrial Revolution created an unprecedented migration of people from the countryside to towns, resulting in rapid urban growth; between 1801 and 1831, Liverpool's population grew from 77,000 to 202,000 and Manchester's from 75,000 to 182,000. The absence of planning or building controls during this period meant that little consideration was given to either population density or the need for adequate drainage and access to clean water. The ensuing insanitary conditions and overcrowding resulted in infectious diseases, such as smallpox, tuberculosis, cholera and typhoid, becoming significant causes of death and morbidity; life expectancy in the worst industrial towns was as low as 19 years.

There was therefore an inevitability about the emergence of epidemics such as cholera and it is likely that the first cholera epidemic of 1831–32, which killed over 22,000 people in England, was a key element in the emergence of the sanitary movement – the forerunner of the public health movement. At this time it was believed that disease was caused by poisonous, foul-smelling vapours from decomposing matter (the 'miasmic' theory). Improved sanitation to remove these smells and hence the source of the disease was considered the solution; a view supported by the observation that cholera was commonest where overcrowding and squalor, and hence smells, were most intense and strongest.

In 1842, Edwin Chadwick, the secretary of the Poor Law Commission, published *The Sanitary Condition of the Labouring Population of Great Britain* describing the appalling conditions under which many people lived. Chadwick, heavily influenced by the Utilitarian philosophy of 'the greatest happiness for the greatest number', argued strongly and passionately that disease could be eliminated if social conditions were changed. Chadwick's report, the emerging sanitary movement and the outbreak of the second cholera epidemic in 1848 were the main drivers for the introduction of the Public Health Act 1848 and the beginning of the modern public health movement.

The Public Health Act 1848 required towns where the death rate was over 23 per 1,000 to establish local Boards of Health responsible for cleansing, adequate water supplies, sewerage, drainage and the regulation of slaughterhouses. The main officers of the board were a surveyor, an officer of health and an inspector of nuisances. Implementation was patchy as the Act was permissive where the death rate was less than 23 per 1,000 and therefore influenced by local attitudes and vested interests. It needed a further two epidemics of cholera and the death of Prince Albert from typhoid to convince the government of the day to introduce the Local Government Act 1872 requiring all districts to provide public health services led by Medical Officers of Health (MOH) and to consolidate all existing public health legislation into the Public Health Act 1875.

The Public Health Act 1875 was important for a number of reasons:

- Local authorities were required to provide public health services such as meat inspection, the provision of water supplies, sewerage, drainage and cleansing and required to regulate and inspect common lodging houses.
- Local authorities had the power to provide hospitals (fever hospitals) and medicines for epidemic control and a variety of powers to control infectious diseases.
- The appointment of an MOH became obligatory.

This Act was a milestone and gave local authorities far-reaching powers to intervene on behalf of the health of their population.

The scientific basis of public health action was strengthened by the work of John Snow, Louis Pasteur and Robert Koch. In 1854, John Snow demonstrated that the pattern of disease in a cholera outbreak in Soho was consistent with infection caused by drinking faecally contaminated water from the Broad Street pump, and not with miasmic transmission. In 1857, Louis Pasteur was able to demonstrate that the toxins thought to cause certain diseases were in fact living organisms and by 1864 had developed the germ theory to explain his findings. Robert Koch provided further support for the germ theory by identifying the bacteria causing tuberculosis in 1882 and cholera in 1884. The debunking of the miasmic theory of disease transmission and the acceptance of the germ theory of disease was a significant step forward in the development of public health; it established the importance of the study of epidemiology and microbiology in public health and was an effective basis for public health action.

The Boer War provided the unlikely stimulus for the next developments in public health; the rejection of over 28 per cent of army volunteers on health grounds in 1900 caused such alarm that a series of measures were introduced to improve the health of children. The 1906 Education (Provision of Meals) Act permitted local authorities to provide school meals and is the basis of the current school meals service. The 1907 Education (Administrative Provision) Act introduced the schools medical service led by the MOH, the aims of which were to ensure all schoolchildren had regular medical examinations in order to identify disease at an early stage. However, since many of the children's ill health problems were present before school age and infant mortality was still very high (it had not improved in the 50 years before 1900), action was directed at improving care during pregnancy and in the period after birth.

Before the 1902 Midwives Act, many midwives were untrained and this Act required midwives to be certified and registered with a Central Midwives Board; the local supervision of registration was the responsibility of the MOH. The importance of health visiting, started in the 1860s by a group of women from Manchester and Salford to encourage higher standards of child care, was recognised in the 1907 Notification of Births Act. This Act encouraged the notification of all births to the MOH so that a trained health visitor could visit the mother; notification became compulsory after 1915.

During the early twentieth century, public health continued to grow and develop as local authorities were delegated more powers: for example the Local Government Act 1929 transferred the functions of the Poor Law Authorities to county and borough councils, as well as responsibility for vaccination, hospitals and other institutions. It would be fair to say that public health was at its most influential from 1930 until the formation of the National Health Service (NHS) in 1948.

The introduction of the NHS saw the transfer of fever hospitals and infirmaries from local government to the health service. The school health service, health visitors, district nurses and social workers remained with the MOH and the development of community services became a priority. During this period, renewed attention was given to the environment with the Clean Air Act 1956, the Noise Abatement Act 1960 and the Control of Pollution Act 1970. The effects of this were most noticeable in the elimination in the early 1970s of the smogs that had affected many large cities.

Following the 1974 reorganisation of the NHS, many of the services associated with the MOH transferred across into the health service, and community medicine emerged as a medical speciality within the NHS. Social services and environmental health services remained within local government, the latter with support from the new community physicians.

Over the next few years, public health went into decline as the new community physicians found themselves increasingly drawn into the problems of acute medical care and the recurring financial problems of the health service. The public health agenda also changed and infectious disease was no longer perceived to be the problem it had been; cancer and heart disease were now the main causes of death and significant morbidity. However, it was two infectious disease incidents – an outbreak of salmonella at Stanley Royd Hospital and legionnaires' disease at Stafford Hospital – which led to the renaissance of public health. The Acheson Report, Independent Enquiry published 1998 attempted to clarify roles and responsibilities in relation to communicable disease and environmental hazards and the other aspects of public health. The term 'public health' was reintroduced and became formalised in health service guidance in 1993.

The 1990s saw a brief resurgence of interest in the concepts of public health but the managerial focus was on hospital activity and waiting times. The eventual demise of health authorities and the establishment of Primary Care Trusts (PCTs) in 2002 should have seen the resurrection of public health, given the emphasis in general practice on prevention and promoting health. Instead, PCTs rapidly became commissioning organisations focused on meeting healthcare targets and many within PCTs questioned the added value of public health. In 2003, the creation of the Health Protection Agency took the leadership, but not the responsibility, for infectious disease and other environmental issues away from the health service, further fragmenting public health in PCTs.

CASE STUDY

Information has been summarized from the Health Protection Agency (HPA) website (www.hpa.org.uk 2008) and typifies the evolving and dynamic focus of public health in the UK and the role of the HPA in the context of current public health issues.

The Agency's roles are 'to protect the community (or any part of the community) against infectious diseases and other dangers to health' (HPA Act 2004). This is provided by the HPA via an integrated approach to protecting UK public health through support and advice to the NHS, local authorities, emergency services and others who also have health protection responsibilities. The Agency was established as a special health authority in 2003 and then as a non-departmental public body in 2005, with radiation protection as part of its remit.

The Agency's services are provided through:

- **The Centre for Emergency Preparedness and Response** – prepares for and co-ordinates responses to potential healthcare emergencies and undertakes basic and applied research into understanding infectious diseases.
- **The Centre for Infections** – includes infectious disease surveillance, providing specialist microbiology and epidemiology services, coordinating

the investigation and cause of national and uncommon outbreaks, helping to advise government on the risks posed by various infections and responding to international health alerts.

- **The HPA Centre for Radiation, Chemical and Environmental Hazards** – comprises the Radiation Protection Division and the Chemical Hazards and Poisons Division.
- **Local and Regional Health Protection Agency services** – work alongside the NHS providing specialist support in communicable disease and infection control, and emergency planning. They also oversee some laboratory services.

The Agency continues to provide a range of specialist services and advice; training doctors, nurses, scientists, emergency services and others in emergency preparedness and response including potential bioterrorist incidents; surveillance of potential threats to public health; works across national and international boundaries to reduce the impact of threats to public health; leads on Port Health arrangements.

CONCLUSION

What does the future hold for public health? There is little doubt that many in power acknowledge and support the public health agenda; public health is now everybody's business but no one's responsibility and there is still a lack of an overall sense of direction. Is the NHS, with its preoccupation with healthcare delivery and targets, the right place for what remains of public health, with its emphasis on promoting health? Local authorities are still responsible for many services that could promote health, education, housing and leisure services; perhaps it is time to capitalise on the move for the director of public health to be a joint local authority and health service appointment?

FURTHER READING

Martin, C., Lewis, E. and Rees, R. (2001) *Poverty and Public Health 1815–1948*. Oxford: Heinemann.

Pencheon, D., Guest, C., Melzer, D. and Muir Gray, J.A. (2006) *The Oxford Handbook of Public Health Practice*, 2nd revised edn. Oxford: Oxford University Press.

key concepts
in public health

2 Modern Public Health

Fiona Adshead and Allison Thorpe

DEFINITION

Public policy has been defined as 'the broad framework of ideas and values within which decisions are taken and action, or inaction, is pursued by governments in relation to some issue or problem' (O'Neill and Pederson, 1992). As such, policy generically can be described as a guiding principle of, not a guarantee for, action. Public health policy more specifically reflects an increasingly diverse agenda, developed against a context of global forces and changing social and political environments. An active social justice agenda and growing evidence of the impact of the social determinants of health on health inequalities and outcomes make more complex an already crowded picture. In this chapter we will look at the implications of current policy drivers in England for public health, with a particular focus on how at a national level policy directions are often influenced by, and influence, legislative frameworks and policies which are enacted at a European or global level.

KEY POINTS

- Public health policy is not designed or delivered in isolation from the social and political context – it is linked to a wide range of social resources and infrastructures, social capital, social interaction and social support.
- Policy boundaries are often blurred – European directives can both limit autonomy of action at a national level and ensure local activity has a resonance over a larger population level by setting clear parameters for action across nation states.
- Modern public health policy and practice has to be able to respond to economic, demographic and epidemiological transitions, while still enabling everyday action on the ground.

modern public health

11

- With lifestyle-related diseases rising, people's expectation of active engagement in promoting and protecting their own health means that the practice of public health is becoming increasingly personalised. This is reflected in the policy arena.

DISCUSSION

Policy-makers working in the field of public health today face a very different environment to that which faced our forebears in the nineteenth century. Then, the primary focus of public health activity centred on sanitation, slum clearance and the prevention of infectious diseases (Gorsky, 2007). In our more modern complex society, we face new challenges. Rising rates of diabetes linked to obesity, escalating chronic diseases, and global tobacco control – to name but a small selection of our concerns – are juxtaposed with an increasingly articulate, educated consumer society and an increasingly engaged media and business presence. Unsurprisingly, against such a backdrop, it has long been remarked that for public health 'boundaries are fiction' (Terry, 1964).

Determining how best to assure the health of our populations remains an enormous agenda – and one in which the whole of society has a shared interest, with roles for government, the healthcare system, the wider population, the community, and business itself. There has been a tangible policy move in recent years towards health improvement initiatives which take a wider partnership approach to delivering on health (DH, 2007d). Reports, such as the eponymous Wanless reports, have been successful in driving home the message that a sustainable healthcare system requires 'full engagement' of the people in its delivery (HM Treasury, 2002, 2004). With recent economic analysis suggesting that the total cost of preventable illness is 19 per cent of total GDP for England (NSMC, 2006), prevention is increasingly seen as the key factor in addressing growing concerns about the affordability of healthcare systems into the future (HM Treasury, 2002, 2004). Successive policy documents, such as *Choosing Health* (DH, 2004a) and *Our Health, Our Care, Our Say* (DH, 2006e) have reinforced this message, reflecting a recognition that no amount of legislation, regulation or structural adjustment can compete with the ability of people to choose how they live their lives. But such a person-centred approach for public health policy is a challenge in itself.

CASE STUDY

The recent smoke-free legislation, which came into effect on 1 July 2007 in England, provides a tangible demonstration of the relationship between politics, policy development, the individual and the evidence. Despite evidence that second-hand smoke was a determinant of ill health, there was considerable resistance to the idea of taking a comprehensive legislative approach to the issue, largely centred around the human rights of smokers. The eventual policy decision to allow an open vote on how to progress the legislation was the culmination of a long campaign, which drew upon:

- policy-driven public consultations;
- high levels of popular and professional support;
- an extensive evidence base;
- examples of local-level action which was considerably ahead of the proposed national policy direction;
- international and, in the case of Scotland and Ireland, more local examples of the success of enacting national legislation in other countries, with Scotland, for example, demonstrating a drop in symptoms in bar workers from 79 per cent to 53 per cent within one month of implementation (Menzies et al., 2006).

The combination of these factors raised the level of debate, and ultimately influenced politicians to vote for the more radical and visionary legislation which was eventually enacted. This reinforces the need to recognise that public health policy cannot be designed or delivered in isolation from the social and political context: political decisions have to reflect a balance between the evidence and public opinion regarding what is right – and both affordable and sustainable – for society at the given point in time. The journey there, and the full engagement which characterised it, critically determines the success of the outcome.

However, the success of the policy direction does not lie solely in the enactment of the legislation, but will be measured by its cumulative effect on the health of the population. In this case, enactment of the legislation is only one manifestation of the policy direction. Alongside this policy-makers are working to build on this historic milestone, through effective enforcement, policing and publicity, to encourage people to take advantage of health improvement initiatives, such as smoking cessation services, which will spare thousands more lives, and through consultations to raise the age of sale, to ensure that more people are spared the misery

13

of watching their families and friends suffer with preventable smoke-related illnesses (DH, 2007a).

This recognition of the need to take a more personalised approach to health underpinned the *Choosing Health* White Paper, reflecting a policy commitment to a broader social contract between the state and individuals, with choice and civic action being key elements of this contract. In effect, it recognised that public health policy needs both to provide a direction for and support action in relation to our key health priorities. In practice this means that policies must facilitate partnership across society, with joined up action at governmental, national, regional and local levels, and enable those who have an ability to contribute to do so. In practice, this means that policy direction must be supported by the appropriate levers to drive delivery:

- realistic shared, cross-government targets which commit governments to improving health outcomes in their population;
- co-ordination across government, and where necessary across national boundaries;
- a commitment to wider action to improve the health of the most disadvantaged and tackle health inequalities, e.g. through action on housing, fuel poverty and employment;
- use of social marketing and other techniques to change social norms.

CONCLUSION

Policy direction in England reflects our understanding that health cannot be imposed on people, nor can we expect them to be co-producers of sustainable good health without support from government. The relationship between public health, the state and the population is complex. Today, more than ever, we need to face up to a complex conundrum:

- Applying policy consistently across nation states sets clear parameters for action and enables local action to have a stronger resonance across a wider population. Legislation provides one route to ensure this, but legislation alone will not deliver behavioural change.
- Working with the population, targeting our efforts appropriately, ensures that the effects of our policy will be instrumental in informing a culture that is motivated, progressive, ambitious and constantly striving to improve services: not for the sake of it or to satisfy 'managers', but for the benefit of service users.

But, as the case study demonstrated, it is not an 'either/or' scenario. Policy-makers today working in the field of public health face a complex agenda – but they also have a unique range of opportunities. It is up to the population as a whole to ensure that we maximise their potential.

FURTHER READING

French J. and Blair S., C. (2006) 'From snake oil salesmen to trusted policy advisors. The development of a strategic approach to the application of social marketing in England', *Social Marketing Quarterly*, 12(3): 29–40.

HM Treasury (2002) *Securing our Future: Taking a Long Term View*. London: HM Treasury.

O'Neill, M. and Pederson, A. (1992) 'Building a methods bridge between policy analysis and healthy public policy', *Canadian Journal of Public Health*, 83(32): 25–30.

World Health Organisation. (2006) *WHO Framework Convention on Tobacco Control*. Retrieved January 21, 2007, from http://www.who.int/fctc/whofctc_cover_english.pdf

World Health Organisation (2007) *Interim Statement of the Commission on Social Determinants of Health 2007*. Retrieved January 21, 2007, from http://www.who.int/social_determinants/resources/interim_statement/en/index.html

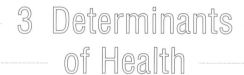

3 Determinants of Health

Soumen Sengupta

DEFINITION

Health is classically defined as 'a state of complete physical, social and mental health, and not merely the absence of disease or infirmity' (WHO, 1948). As such, health is as much a social construct as a biological characteristic. It is the product of a complex interaction of different factors: this is true at both individual and population levels. These determinants include not just an individual's particular characteristics and behaviours but also their economic, physical and social environments (Ashton and Seymour, 1992).

KEY POINTS

- Health is created by a complicated interaction of different factors, only some of which can be directly influenced by individuals.
- Social determinants tend to have a greater impact on population health status than healthcare services.
- Different determinants have a differential influence on different groups of people: this can contribute to health inequalities.
- An appreciation of the differential influence of determinants should be used to develop and deploy a wider array of public policy activities to promote good health.

DISCUSSION

How different disciplines consider determinants of health is born of their traditions and values. There are four schools of thought (Beaglehole, 2004):

- The biomedical view – emphasis on specific causes and discrete treatments for ill health amongst individuals.
- The lifestyle view – emphasis on individual responsibility for lifestyle choices.
- The broad socio-economic approach – emphasis on factors outside the healthcare sector, especially economic and social.
- The population health view – emphasis on the impact on population health of wealth generation and distribution.

Whilst the biomedical view has traditionally dominated health policy, recent years have seen increasing recognition of a more comprehensive suite of determinants (HM Treasury, 2004). Although healthcare services have some impact, more influential on population health are the economic, physical and social conditions that foster ill health – and that, if orientated correctly, should actively engender good health (Ashton and Seymour, 1992).

Developing a comprehensive perspective

Canada's Lalonde Report was the first official statement to describe a broader view of health (Lalonde, 1974). Its 'health field' concept described how health status was not just affected by biology and health-care services, but was explicitly a product of lifestyle behaviours and the environment. This was then developed, most prominently in the Ottawa Charter for Health Promotion (WHO, 1984) which set out nine pre-requisites for good health:

- Peace
- Shelter
- Education
- Food
- Income
- A stable ecosystem
- Sustainable resources
- Social justice
- Equity

Consequently, an ambitious proposition has been developed for priori-tising resources 'upstream', from services targeted at the individual to policy action on the economic, physical and social determinants of pop-ulation health. Unfortunately, most investment in health still reflects and reinforces the biomedical worldview (Hunter, 2003).

Social determinants of health

Systems theory states that a system is composed of interdependent and interrelated parts, with change in one part producing changes in others (von Bertalanffy, 1968). In order to explore the impacts of and the potential to influence different determinants it is thus necessary to appreciate their interrelationships. A number of conceptual models assist this. The most frequently cited is the Dahlgren and Whitehead 'rainbow' – Figure 3.1 (Dahlgren and Whitehead, 1991).

The extent to which different determinants can be influenced varies; certainly no individual is likely to exert direct control over most of them. Furthermore, these determinants can have a differential impact at different stages of an individual's life; between different social groups; and between different countries (Solar and Irwin, 2007). Clearly con-text is crucial.

Much of the discussion on determinants within the public health arena has focused on social factors. The rationale is that, however impor-tant individual genetic susceptibilities to disease may be, population health has been influenced much more by the rapidly changing social

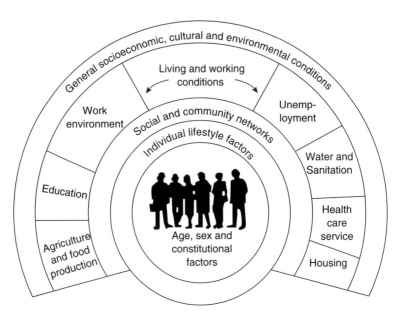

Figure 3.1   *Dahlgren and Whitehead's determinants of health model (1991)*

conditions in which people live (WHO, 2003). By focusing on social determinants, Graham and Kelly (2004) has suggested that different models implicitly follow a common structure that articulates a causal chain between the wider environmental elements and health status.

That said, it is important to recognise the value of healthcare interventions in reducing disease susceptibility (e.g. immunisation programmes). It is also important to remember that wider environmental factors should not be viewed as disconnected from the experiences of individuals. Simply put, these social systems are a product of individuals and their interactions. Moreover, the choices that individuals make should not be dismissed. However, they are a product of the choices available and the confidence different groups have in exercising them (i.e. the degree of self-efficacy possessed). Circumstances and conditions that provide people with greater control over different facets of their lives (and consequently nurture a greater sense of self-esteem) are associated with better health outcomes (Marmot, 2003).

Health inequalities

Consideration of the differential influences of health determinants is almost inextricably linked to the question of why economically or socially disadvantaged groups consistently experience relatively poorer health status (Graham and Kelly, 2004). Such disadvantage can manifest in different forms, e.g. limited aspirations, low income and discrimination. Critically, such disadvantages tend to gravitate towards one another, creating vicious circles in which people get trapped.

In the UK, the Black Report (Townsend et al., 1992) identified the primary reasons for worsening social gradients in mortality and other indicators of ill health as material deprivation and poverty; and its recommendations highlighted economic and social policy solutions. These conclusions were reinforced by subsequent publications, with the Acheson Report (Acheson, 1998) stating that: 'the weight of scientific evidence supports a socio-economic explanation of health inequalities. This traces the roots of ill health to such determinants as income, education and employment as well as material environment and lifestyle.' While there are clearly overlaps, the determinants of health are not exactly the same as the determinants of health inequality: the latter concerns the unequal (and by implication, unfair) distribution of health determinants (Graham and Kelly, 2004).

CASE STUDY

Understanding determinants should help identify different policy levers (local, regional, national and transnational) that can promote health amongst different communities. This could include action to develop resilience amongst young people and vulnerable adults; strengthen social capital; improve infrastructure and access to services; and tighten environmental legislation. It should enable identification and mitigation of policy action that could have a detrimental impact – this is the essence of health impact assessment (Brown et al., 2005). It should also help develop a realistic sense of the limitations of any given intervention to improve population health. For example, although statins are a relatively effective pharmacological intervention for reducing the risk of heart disease (NICE, 2006), against the backdrop of an escalating obesity epidemic they can only have a limited impact in themselves (WHO, 2007). That does not mean they are not worth providing, but rather that they need to be part of a multi-dimensional package of activities.

Cross-references

Understanding health determinants has relevance to all aspects of public health. In using this textbook, it would be particularly useful to cross-reference with inequalities in health (Chapter 5); assessing public health need (Chapter 21); planning public health initiatives (Chapter 22); health impact assessment (Chapter 24); and collaborative and partnership working (Chapter 34).

CONCLUSION

Health at both individual and population levels is the product of a complicated interaction of different factors. Health policy is still dominated by a biomedical paradigm, yet there is a substantial theoretical and evidence base to support a more comprehensive perspective. It is now widely understood that the primary determinants of health are the economic, physical and social environments within which individuals live. Few determinants can be directly influenced by the individual; and most social determinants have a greater impact on population health status than healthcare services. Critically, many determinants have a differential impact on different groups of people: this can contribute to inequalities in health. Developing an understanding of the complex nature of the health determinants is not a merely theoretical exercise; nor should the recognition of that complexity act as an excuse for inaction on discrete issues. Rather this understanding should be used to develop and deploy a wider array of public policy activities to promote good health.

FURTHER READING

Irwin, A. and Scali, E. (2005) *Action on the Social Determinants of Health: Learning from Previous Experiences*. Geneva: World Health Organization.

Kelly, M., Bonnefoy, J., Morgan, A. and Florenzano, F. (2006) *The Development of the Evidence Base about the Social Determinants of Health*. Geneva: World Health Organization.

key concepts
in public health

4 Public Health Theories

Ann Bryan

DEFINITION

A theory is the articulation of the framework of beliefs and knowledge which enable us to explain a specific phenomenon. One of the major problems for public health practitioners is that theories are not articulated in everyday language but are made up of concepts and constructs which are often difficult to understand. Perhaps this is one reason why some commentators have argued that theories are unnecessary and need to be eradicated and replaced by common sense or professional judgement (Pring, 2000). However, the practical understanding which underpins common sense and professional judgement is built on assumptions and lacks the validity and truth of theoretical explanations. It is the theoretical perspective which informs research methodology and provides a context for its logic and criteria.

Defining public health theory is a complex issue. As a term, it is used in a variety of contexts according to the knowledge base of the occupational group promoting public health. For example, biomedicine, psychology, social policy and education all bring different theoretical interpretations to the subject. It has even been suggested that public health is atheoretical in the sense that practice has been largely unaffected by the explicit application of theory (Weed, 2002). Indeed, Wills and Earle (2007: 129) state it is possible to promote public health 'without any knowledge, or understanding, of the theory that underpins practice', although they do not believe this will lead to effective strategies.

This chapter aims to review the value and limitations of the traditional theory base of public health. It will also highlight the potential importance of current emerging theories in public health research and their implications for promoting effective practice. As public health practitioners have an obligation to act in the best interests of the population they are serving, it is vital that all theories underpinning knowledge and practice are given due consideration.

KEY POINTS

- Public health theory is a dynamic process.
- Public health theory has been influenced by chronological eras, distinguished by dominant theories.
- Public health theory has important implications for public health strategy and application to practice.

DISCUSSION

The development of public health theory is evolutionary in nature. It has always reflected different chronological eras which are defined by their prevailing paradigms, research methods and preventative practices (Nicolau et al., 2007). These eras have been categorised by Susser and Susser in the epidemiological literature (1996a) as the sanitary movement era, the germ theory era and the chronic disease era. Current developments in public health theory suggest that a fourth era has now emerged (March and Susser 2006).

Sanitary movement era

Public health has its roots in the sanitary movement which gained strength during the first half of the nineteenth century and was based on the miasma theory of disease causation. Miasma theorists believed that decomposing organic matter created harmful odours and particles within the atmosphere which contributed to the development of disease.

Hence, public health measures to a large extent were concerned with sanitation. The focus was on disease prevention and the health needs of the total population. The sanitary reforms brought about major health improvements even though the underlying theory was inaccurate. At this time epidemiology, centring on the causes of disease in populations, was truly a part of public health and public health practitioners were largely involved in population-wide health improvements (Susser and Susser, 1996a).

Germ theory era

Germ theory was the foremost theory in public health science from the latter half of the nineteenth century until at least the mid-twentieth century. Following the discovery of bacteria, laboratory-based diagnosis, immunisation and treatment gradually marginalised miasma theory. The dominant paradigm moved from being population-based to being focused on disease pathology and the treatment of individuals. This analysis became even more ascendant with the growth of the medical-industrial complex which, as MacDonald (2004: 384) states, 'cemented the biomedical emphasis on single-causative agents' and led to the weakening of population-based public health with the centralisation of power and resources in hospital-based services. Epidemiology became a derivative activity rather than a creative science in its own right as it had been earlier.

Chronic disease era

By the mid-twentieth century infectious-disease mortality had started to decline in the industrialised world and much more consideration was given to other causes of disease. This led to a corresponding decline in germ theory and the evolution of a new epidemiological paradigm which came to be known as the 'risk factor' or 'black box' paradigm (Susser and Susser, 1996b). The fundamental premise of this paradigm is that chronic disease is multi-causal and cannot be explained by a specific factor. Some of the theory's leading proponents accepted the need for a multi-professional approach and specified populations as the sample of investigation. However, in general, chronic disease epidemiology has centred on individual personal behaviour and has often failed to consider the wider public health agenda (Pearce, 1996).

Current theoretical trends

Contemporary public health theory appears to be polarising. One move is towards the micro level of molecular and genetic epidemiology and the other is towards a broader, macro level social perspective described by some commentators as social epidemiology (Saracci, 1999; Susser, 1999; Krieger, 2001).

Biological technology has altered the way in which disease is understood at the micro level. It is popular with the public as it gives definite solutions to identifiable problems. However, the research methods and preventative practices involved in biological techniques are extremely expensive and may not necessarily have a global impact.

According to Krieger (2001), there are three main social epidemiological theories: psychosocial, social production of disease/political economy of health, and ecosocial. These theories illuminate **principles which attempt to give reasons** for the social inequalities in health and disease distribution. They argue that health and disease are the consequence of social, political, environmental, fiscal and demographic causes. Where they diverge is in the weight they allocate to 'different aspects of social and biological conditions in shaping population health, how they integrate social and biological explanations, and thus their recommendations for action' (Krieger, 2001: 669). Psychosocial and social production of disease/political economy of health theories, place little emphasis on the biological process, whereas the ecosocial paradigm grants it due recognition.

Ecosocial theory accepts the holistic notion that individual human beings, societal structures, the environment and biology are mutually significant in formulating patterns of health, wellbeing and disease in the total population (MacDonald, 2004). This multi-level paradigm offers inter-disciplinary, public health practitioners a way forward with its new methodologies and practices. Its defining characteristics are not only the environmental standpoint but also the social concepts of collaboration and community participation. Hence, ecosocial theory can provide a practitioner with the knowledge base to devise strategies which will impact on the delivery of effective public health practice.

CASE STUDY

Margaret is the health visitor for an isolated, council-owned, traveller site which has recently been vandalised and is in an insanitary condition. She is the key contact for the traveller families and visits them regularly. One of her clients is Carla, a 26-year-old mother, who lives on benefits in a caravan. She is overweight, suffers from depression and smokes at least 40 cigarettes a day. Her father died at 45 from a heart attack and her mother has a chronic chest condition. She has four children. Mary, aged 7, and Danny, aged 6, have not received a regular education, while Jade and Thomas, who are both under 3, are behind in their development. Furthermore, all the family and many other site dwellers are suffering from impetigo.

Margaret, drawing on her knowledge of contemporary, ecosocial, public health theory, calls a multi-agency meeting, including traveller representatives, to discuss the public health issues relating to the above circumstances. As a result of this consultation, the agencies and the site community are able to secure financial support for the upgrading of sanitary facilities and organise transport to enable the children to attend school. Furthermore, they succeed in improving access to medical and social amenities for all site members. By viewing health, disease and wellbeing from an ecosocial perspective, Margaret has formulated an effective public health strategy at the individual, community and environmental levels.

CONCLUSION

Public health theory is constantly evolving and will continue to play an important part in promoting effective practice. As outlined above, dominant paradigms have been superseded as health patterns and technologies have changed (Susser and Susser, 1996a). In the last decade there has been a move in the level of analysis from the individual back towards the population. This has resulted in new methodologies and practices which are reflected in the more diverse and comprehensive nature of inter-disciplinary public health which dominates our modern era.

FURTHER READING

Naidoo, J. and Wills, J. (2005) *Public Health and Health Promotion: Developing Practice*, 2nd edn. Edinburgh: Ballière, Tindall.
Earle, S., Lloyd, C. E., Sidell, M. and Spurr, S. (2007) *Theory and Research in Promoting Public Health*. London: Sage.

5 Inequalities in Health

Nicola Close

DEFINITION

Despite improving health across the country over many generations there is still a large variation in health status, life expectancy, mortality and morbidity between different groups of people. Much of this is avoidable and unfair, and should more accurately be described as health inequity: an unjust distribution of health and healthcare. These differences in health outcomes are known as health inequalities.

Why should a boy born in Kensington expect on average to live around eight years longer than one born in Manchester?

The reduction of these unfair inequalities should be the public health practitioner's and commissioner's aim.

KEY POINTS

- Many health inequalities are avoidable.
- Inequalities are assessed in a variety of powerful ways, but the mapping used does not show causes or solutions.
- The gap between the healthiest and unhealthiest is a gradient and not a clear-cut division between healthy and unhealthy.
- A multi-agency partnership approach is essential to tackle all the determinants.

DISCUSSION

Looking at inequalities in health is not a modern interest. Since at least the 1840s there have been reports monitoring differences in health. Social and public health reformers from Chadwick to Beveridge have used evidence of a health gap to back their reforms. The Black Report (Black, 1980) is widely regarded as the turning point in national attempts to explain inequalities and link policy and action to decrease them. However, the change in government before its publication meant that Black's report lay unactioned, and it was not until 1997 that another report was commissioned. This Acheson Inquiry (1998) led to the current emphasis on reducing health inequalities as a key target both for government and locally.

In the years since then there has been real progress in measuring inequalities. Key national and local targets have been set for achieving a reduction and there have been numerous policy initiatives (DH, 2003). However, it is clear that raising the profile has not been matched by a fall in the gap between the healthiest and unhealthiest in our society.

When the political will is there, why is it so difficult to achieve equity?

Assessment and mapping

The mapping of health outcomes across geographical areas (e.g. Welsh Assembly Govt, 2006) and also for specific groups of people (e.g.

Association of public health observatories, 2005) is routinely carried out by information analysts and epidemiologists. More complex statistical measures are used to describe the health gap (e.g. Eastern Regional Public Health Observatories, 2006): these help to monitor whether inequality is increasing or decreasing over time.

All these pictures can give a powerful illustration of where health inequalities exist and are enormously useful for gaining support and resources for action, but they are generally uninformative about how to address the health differences.

The lack of progress then does not lie with the assessment of inequalities.

Causes and interventions

The scientific evidence has established that poverty and uneven distribution of resources account for the larger part of health inequalities (see Chapter 14). The more deprived the population, the poorer the health outcome. This has been shown repeatedly regarding heart disease, mental health, cancers or indeed most health, wellbeing and illness measures.

However, poverty alone does not cause illness. The reasons for health inequalities range across the spectrum of determinants of health; economic, social, psychological and environmental factors interact with personal behaviours and access to care. This complex picture has to be reflected in a multi-faceted approach to tackling inequality.

For instance, unemployment, isolation and poor housing could interact with addictive personality to produce poor health caused by alcohol abuse. The existence of preventative and care services is unlikely to ensure complete take-up of those services by individuals while short-term relief from the difficulties of living is a higher priority than longer-term health outcomes.

The corollary of the scenario above is that those who have a more comfortable life are more likely to take up the opportunities for improved health outcomes that are available. Blanket coverage of service provision is then likely to lead to an increase in the health gap, with the better off and better educated using the services disproportionately. Thus the cycle of increasing provision has led over the last century to vastly improved health overall in the UK whilst health inequalities have increased.

Successful action on inequalities should therefore be based on joined up approaches between the Local Strategic Partnership agencies.

Government initiatives such as Local Area Agreements are helpful approaches to facilitate the multi-agency partnership.

Health equity audit

What is needed then is: an accurate and appropriate assessment; an evidence-based approach to what works in terms of improving health outcomes; and partnership working to ensure that all the determinants are covered in a comprehensive and cohesive programme.

A newer assessment tool aiming to do just that, and which is becoming the must-do for assessing and addressing inequalities, is the Health Equity Audit (ERPHO, 2002). This compares need (using a health indicator) with a matched service provision across groups. Where this mapping shows discrepancies between provision and need, this should be addressed.

Targeting

It was established earlier in this chapter that the right intervention may improve health, but often at the expense of widening the health gap. Perhaps then the answer is to target provision to those groups of people with the poorest health. There are several problems that arise with this approach.

The first is that there is not a clear split between the haves and have-nots. There is a gradient in health outcomes in any population, often matched by the social gradient of deprivation. Ideally, provision should follow the reverse pattern of this gradient. However this would mean providing a shifting pattern of service, which is impracticable. In practice, any decision to target will have to draw an artificial line to say who gets the provision and who does not. Filtering a population along these lines is never easy and often gives rise to complex bureaucracy and injustices. Think, for instance about means-tested benefits.

An easier route is to target specific geographical areas, which often equate to the most deprived areas. This is the basis for a lot of the work around health and social exclusion. But it is not without problems. Paradoxically, most poor people do not live in deprived areas (although the risk of being poor is greater in deprived areas than elsewhere). Indeed it could be argued that being poor in an affluent area could mean that you are more deprived than if you live in a poorer area.

So one problem is that targeting deprived areas will only reach the minority of those we would want to reach and so will have a limited effect. Finally, targeting can be stigmatising (think of free school meals) and there are issues about uptake and maintaining the quality of services wholly targeted at the deprived.

CASE STUDY: SURE START

Sure Start is a government programme, launched in 1998 by the Treasury with the aim of delivering the best start in life for every child and bringing together early education, childcare, health and family support. The programmes were originally based in the most deprived areas catering for *all* children up to 4 years old within that area, thus reducing any associated stigma. They were community led with local autonomy for provision, with advice that services must be evidence based.

In its review of the impact of the programme (NESS, 2005) the National Evaluation of Sure Start Local Programmes (SSLP) found several worrying effects in relation to inequalities. Most notably:

> those from *relatively* less (but still) disadvantaged households residing in SSLP areas benefit somewhat from living in these areas...
>
> In contrast, within these same deprived communities, children from *relatively* more disadvantaged families (i.e. teen mother, lone parent, workless household) appear to be adversely affected by living in a SSLP community.

Other concerns raised in local evaluations were about very deprived children living outside programme areas who were unable to access the provision: as we noted above, these comprise most of the deprived children in the country.

This exemplifies both of the key problems associated with interventions aimed at reducing inequalities: any universal intervention will tend to benefit most those least in need of it, thus increasing inequalities; and this is true across any population, however narrowly defined. Any targeted intervention will tend to exclude many of those who would benefit most from it, as well as being liable to stigma and a reduction in quality.

It could be argued that the most effective step is designing access around those who are most in need.

CONCLUSION

We must ensure that we are preventing further inequalities while tackling those that already exist. Undertaking Health Inequality Impact Assessments in advance of policy implementation across all the public sector would go some way towards this goal.

FURTHER READING

Carr-Hill, R. and Chalmers-Dixon, P. (2005) *The Public Health Observatory Handbook of Health Inequalities Measurement.* Oxford: SEPHO.
Whitehead, M., Townsend, P. and Davidson, N. (1992) *Inequalities in Health: The Black Report and the Health Divide.* London: Penguin.

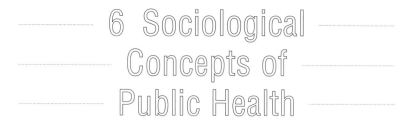

6 Sociological Concepts of Public Health

Dr Andy Lovell

DEFINITION

Three particular strands of health policy contributing towards the emergence of the 'new regime of total health' have become prominent in recent decades: community rather than hospital care, the rise of consumerism and the impact of health promotion and the 'new' public health (Armstrong, 1993). This chapter describes the sociological contribution to the third of these strands and comprises three elements: the risk society context coupled with sociological critiques of the 'new' public health and health promotion. Sociology provides a critical apparatus for examining the societal conditions that have facilitated a new discourse surrounding the relationship between the state and the health of its citizens. These conditions include escalating risk underpinned by the 1970s critique of curative medicine; the subsequent 'new' public health movement never fully responded to concern about 'victim blaming' or how it differed from what came earlier.

KEY POINTS

- Social change over the last few decades has witnessed a context of increased risk, multiple lifestyle choices, and individuals having to adapt to conditions of constant uncertainty.
- Healthcare may be responding to changes by reducing the emphasis on individual care and looking at the management of populations sharing health characteristics.
- The 'new' public health heralded a new era of combining individual responsibility with renewed emphasis on the environment.
- Sociological thought can be employed in an analysis of the health promotion project itself and how it might account for dimensions of social difference.

DISCUSSION

The risk society context

Giddens (1991) and Beck (1992) argued that a new climate of risk was emerging as liberal democracies grappled with the vicissitudes of globalisation and late industrialisation. Escalating world environmental deterioration contributed to conditions of uncertainty, with individual decision-making and calculations of the self becoming increasingly complex and bound by a context of risk. Late modern culture, characterised by a 'politics of anxiety' (Turner, 1991: 24), involved multiple lifestyle options, declining tradition, increased choice and unpredictability, the response to which must be the reconstitution of the self according to the endemic nature of crisis (Giddens, 1991). Beck (1992) discusses the individual's estrangement from traditional mechanisms of social class and the nuclear family in informing lifestyle choice, arguing that different forms of consumer and work-related dependencies are emerging in accordance with market, fashion and policy pressures. Individuals must make decisions according to calculations of risk and opportunity, shaping their own biography, identity, appearing to be in control of one's own destiny.

Castel (1991) takes a different approach, derived from Foucault, elaborating on the idea of risk as political technology and, specifically, the role of expertise in the administration of populations. He envisages a revolution in healthcare characterised by the end of the practitioner–patient relationship, with health professionals absorbed in health strategy and population profiling, and the consequent marginalisation of non-consumers. Medical professional concerns about diagnosis and prescribing treatment cautiously sought to prevent 'dangerousness', but would increasingly be replaced by the management of individual characteristics, 'risk factors', by the 'epidemiological clinic'. As Castel puts it, 'a risk does not arise from the presence of particular precise danger embodied in a concrete individual or group. It is the effect of a combination of abstract *factors* which render more or less probable the occurrence of undesirable modes of behaviour' (1991: 287, emphasis in original). The key medical role becomes the assessment and subsequent identification of the most effective patient pathway; populations are managed according to age, gender, sexuality, occupation and social class, risk factors that underpin treatment strategy. Practitioners become secondary to administrators, the emerging health strategists in control of resources, manpower, information technology and, ultimately, all clinical decision-making apparatus.

The emergence of the 'new' public health

The rationale of health promotion as the central tenet of the 'new' public health movement is a commitment to a broader socio-structural approach than the more conventional health education strategies (Martin and McQueen, 1989). The 'new' public health movement emerged during the 1970s, a period characterised by questioning of the efficacy and social costs of medicine and the emergence of social movements advocating human rights and improved living conditions. There were influential critiques of conventional biomedicine about the success of surgery and immunization (McKeown, 1976), illustrations of the complicity of medicine in the perpetuation of illness (Illich, 1976), and recognition of the role of capitalism as the main contributor to widespread poor health (Navarro, 1976). The 'new' public health is often portrayed as a reaction against both the curative approach to medicine and the individualistic, sometimes victim-blaming nature of health education, some seeing it as a return to the environmental basis of the movement in the nineteenth century (Young and Whitehead, 1993). Ashton and Seymour (1992) defined the 'new' public health as 'bring[ing] together environmental change and personal preventative measures with appropriate therapeutic interventions' underpinned by a recognition of the social aspects of health problems caused by lifestyles (1992: 21). There is a hierarchy of action, with self-care and responsibility for one's health considered the most important strategies for improving public health, and healthcare delivery constituting an expensive safety net once other approaches have been exhausted. Critics argue that such a preventative emphasis is about the conservation and appropriate use of healthcare resources rather than minimising sickness and discomfort (Lupton, 1995). Even the focus of the World Health Organization, so influential in instigating the movement, was that global health improvement should be for the purpose of people leading socially and economically productive lives (WHO, 1985). The economic concerns of the early public health movement, therefore, continue to influence public discourse, despite the rhetoric which makes it difficult to clearly differentiate 'new' from 'old'.

Sociology applied to health promotion

Thorogood (1992) differentiates the application of sociology to health promotion, whereby it helps to refine and develop practices and techniques, from the sociology of health promotion, a critical analysis of its very assumptions. The first extends the health promotion project, analysing power, emphasising the importance of dimensions of social difference and investigating lay health beliefs. It was based partly on a critique of health education, the complex relationship between behavioural change, adequacy of information provision and the structural dimensions of social action (Bunton, et al., 1991). The concept of empowerment was promoted: this acknowledges issues of gender, class, disability and 'race', particularly emphasising social and political awareness in facilitating individual decision-making. Lay health beliefs were acknowledged by recognition that non-professionals do not passively accept nutritional advice; furthermore, such beliefs are more consistent with the complexity of epidemiology than the simplicity of the health promotion message (Davison et al., 1991). This raises significant concerns about the factual basis and anticipated extent of the information provided in relation to the physiological complexity of the relationship between, for example, cholesterol and heart disease.

The second approach offers a critique of issues of structure and agency, ideology, structural discrimination, social regulation and empowerment. It revolves around social control under advanced capitalism and implicates health promotion workers as a mechanism of regulation. Armstrong (1995), for example, argues that such workers are unwittingly embroiled in the sphere of public surveillance, personified by the medical gaze, as communities replace individuals in the control of health. This is an elaboration of Foucault's (1991) principle of 'governmentality', whereby self-surveillance masquerades as empowerment, the state retreating from welfare provision in favour of individual responsibility and self-regulation, new identities constructed around 'technologies of the self'. Bourdieu (1984) offers an alternative perspective based on lifestyle choices and consumption patterns in relation to goods, leisure and culture, and how these inform the construction of particular types of social distinction and differentiation. The relationship between the expansion of health products and services in capitalist society and the erosion of the boundaries between public health promotion and private sector consumption is of central importance from this viewpoint. Bourdieu discusses 'new cultural intermediaries', exemplified by health promotion workers, who advocate the superiority of certain lifestyles. The current crisis of working-class health, however, surrounding obesity, smoking and alcohol consumption, illustrates the successful promotion of dangerous levels of consumption coupled with the failure to sell the middle-class lifestyle.

CASE STUDY

Melissa is a 35-year-old woman with a mild learning disability, who has lived semi-independently with two other women in a residential area of a small town for the past seven years, in one of a network of houses provided by social services. She lived at home with her parents prior to this. The house is staffed by one support worker for busy periods of the day and at other times the service users cater to their own needs. They sometimes eat together, usually when there is a member of staff around, while at other times they eat separately. Melissa's increasingly indulgent lifestyle has meant that she has gained considerable weight over the last couple of years, which is beginning to affect her health. She is spending less and less time physically active, attending a day centre four mornings a week but doing very little for the rest of her time. A risk assessment, conducted when Melissa first moved in, identified her abilities, concluded that she should be encouraged to take control of her life, but perhaps didn't fully account for the complications of living independently today.

Melissa has a reasonable dietary awareness, differentiating foods regarded as of poor nutritional value, particularly microwave meals, from those, such as fruit and vegetables, generally considered to promote health. Her main problem relates to eating too much, especially packets of biscuits or cakes when she feels under too much pressure. The nurse responsible for health promotion for people with learning disabilities in the locality has assisted in providing information on dietary awareness, believing that it is then the responsibility of the individual to make decisions based on the information provided. Melissa has acquired skills in cooking and food preparation at the Further Education College she attends twice weekly, and does regularly prepare her own meals. The difficulty surrounds balancing the expectation that Melissa should increasingly take control of her own life against the risks of overindulging that characterise consumer society. The sociology of health promotion would suggest that Melissa's learning disability is likely to complicate her relationship with her own health, particularly in relation to making healthy lifestyle choices in the face of multiple images of unhealthy but attractive alternatives.

CONCLUSION

The 'new' public health movement with health promotion at its core has gathered pace over the recent years, but has always attracted criticism in relation to whether it seriously provided something different to earlier movements or addressed the concerns about 'victim' blaming inherent in the previous emphasis on individual reliance.

FURTHER READING

Bartley, M., Blane, D. and Davey-Smith, G. (2000) *The Sociology of Health Inequalities*. Oxford: Blackwell.

Nettleton, S. (2006) *The Sociology of Health and Illness*, 2nd edn. Chichester: Wiley and Son.

Roger, A. and Pilgrim, D. (2005) *A Sociology of Mental Health and Illness*, 3rd edn. Maidenhead: Open University Press.

7 Principles
of Epidemiology

Hamed A. Adetunji

DEFINITION

Epidemiology is the scientific way to study the occurrence as well as the causes of disease or health-related events in the population. It is the basic science underpinning public health and other clinical investigations. According to Last (2007), epidemiology is defined as 'the study of the distribution and determinants of health-related states or events in specified populations and the application of this study to control of health problems'.

KEY POINTS

Epidemiology:

- measures disease frequency to quantify it;
- assesses disease distribution to answer 'to whom', 'where' and 'when' disease occurs;
- identifies what determines who gets or does not get disease.

DISCUSSION

Epidemiology is central to the development of public health practice. Its application in public health includes: to assess the need for healthcare services in the community; to investigate the trends (in health and health determinants); to find out what risk factors are responsible for certain diseases and to identify the protective factors for such diseases (Memon, 2006); to gather information for evidence-based decision-making; to understand and control outbreaks, to understand the threats to health and new issues emerging and to plan policies and programmes (for managing health risks). Other applications include preventing and controlling infectious diseases; understanding the impact of therapeutic intervention; and evaluating preventive and therapeutic programmes.

For example, in order to be able to provide adequate services for diabetic patients in the community, an idea of how many people in the community are diabetic at a point in time (known as the prevalence of diabetes) will be useful. This will enable the policy-makers to make an informed decision on how many healthcare staff trained in the care of diabetes will be needed in such community. This will also affect the decision on whether the current equipment will be enough to cope with the number of diabetic patients. In order to plan for future care for diabetic patients in that community the number of people likely to become diabetic over a given number of years, 'known as the incidence', needs to be ascertained. Knowledge of the incidence of diabetes in this community will therefore be required, together with the prevalence already known, so that future care services for diabetic patients can be planned. Defining incidence and prevalence terms will enhance the understanding of the concept being discussed. Incidence of a disease (or health-related state) is the measure of the rate at which new cases of the disease or health-related event occur in a population during a specified period of time. Put mathematically, it is the:

$$\frac{\text{Number of new cases}}{\text{Population at risk} \times \text{time during which cases were ascertained}}$$

Prevalence of a disease (or health related state) is the proportion of a population that have the disease (or health-related state) at a point in time. This includes both old and new cases.

Epidemiology as a tool for selection of the best delivery method of preventive and curative interventions is another important use of epidemiological studies. Treatment that is most cost-effective for a particular disease condition can be identified using epidemiological techniques. For example, Shipp et al. (1999) conducted a study that focused on testing the cost-effectiveness of personal responsibility against five specific outcomes: glucose control, blood pressure control, lipoprotein control, foot care, and eye care in diabetes management. Fendrick et al. (1992) conducted a study the aim of which was to examine the cost-effectiveness of screening and treatment of diabetic retinopathy among insulin-dependent diabetes mellitus (IDDM) patients in Sweden relative to no screening. The result showed that screening for and treating patients with retinopathy can provide a cost saving of 22–37 million SEK, and 2,300–3,200 sight years can be saved if patients comply with the screening recommendations.

Studies in epidemiology

Epidemiological studies are classified into two broad areas known as observational studies and experimental studies. While the observational studies allow nature to take its course (the investigator measures but does not intervene), in experimental studies the investigator intervenes by giving treatment to change the disease determinant.

Observational studies can either be descriptive or analytical. Descriptive (observational) epidemiology is the most basic. It answers such questions as 'who', 'what', 'where' and 'when' of health-related state occurrence. Descriptive study is one of the first things to carry out: for example on arrival at the scene of an outbreak. This can be in form of a simple description of the health status of a population, which can be based either on routinely available data or special surveys.

Analytical epidemiology on the other hand is concerned with the conduction and analysis of studies to measure if there are possible relationships/associations between potential risk factors and health outcomes. It attempts to answer such questions as 'why' the disease or health-related event happens. Studies that use analytical epidemiology include ecological studies that frequently form the basis of research. These involve studying populations/groups and not individuals.

Cross-sectional studies involve identifying a defined population at a particular point in time and measuring a set of variables individually. These are also known as snapshot studies in that they investigate the population being studied at that point in time. They measure the prevalence of disease and can also measure exposure and effect at the same time.

Case-control studies are frequently used to examine the cause of disease (especially rare diseases). The design will include people with the disease and a control group that matches the group with the disease except that they are free from the disease. Both groups are then compared to check for the presence of the likely cause of the disease.

In cohort studies, people who are free from the disease under investigation are recruited at the beginning of the study. They are then grouped into two: those who are exposed to the potential cause of the disease and those who are not. The two groups are then followed up and occurrence of the disease is compared in the two groups.

Experimental epidemiology applies to studies in which human subjects are used for experiments, and as such it is compulsory to obtain ethical approval before conducting such studies (Last, 2007). There is an experimental group and a control group. The experimental group will have the intervention being measured while the control group will have nothing, or another type of intervention. At the end of the study, the outcome in the experimental and control group is assessed to measure the effects of the intervention given. There are three types:

- *Randomised control trial*: used to investigate a new preventive or therapeutic intervention;
- *Field trial*: as opposed to clinical trials, this is carried out on individuals who, although free from the disease at the beginning of the study, are considered to be at risk of developing it;
- *Community trial*: this is carried out using community as opposed to individual as the subject of the study. It is used to investigate diseases that originate in social conditions.

CASE STUDY

Mr Wale, a public health director applied to the Ministry of Health for a grant to implement a diabetic preventive initiative. He is aware of the fact that knowledge of the group at risk of a particular disease will assist in the planning of prevention or control of such disease, so he targeted obese people in his community. The Minister of Health (before committing money to this project) asked for evidence that obesity is a predisposing factor to developing type 2 diabetes mellitus. In order to have strong evidence for this claim, Mr Wale decides to investigate by carrying out a study. He therefore decided on an observational study design – cohort studies in which a group of individuals that are obese and another group that are not are observed for a number of years. He ensures that the two groups are identical, except that one group is obese and another group is of normal weight. After the end of the study follow-up, the number who became diabetic in each group were counted and the two groups were then compared. He was able to find a link between obesity and diabetes in that more people who were obese were found to be diabetic than those of normal weight who became diabetic during the study. He therefore used the evidence to support the proposed diabetic preventive programme directed at the obese people of his community. The Minister provided the grant for the programme due to evidence from the study. Similar study designs have also been used to establish the fact that people who do not exercise are likely to suffer diabetes, especially type 2 diabetes, whereas physically active people are at lower risk of developing type 2 diabetes. So, if a preventive initiative is to be planned for type 2 diabetes, it can be directed towards encouraging people to be more active so as to reduce the risk of progressing from pre-diabetes to type 2 diabetes (Dunstan et al., 2003).

CONCLUSION

Epidemiology is a discipline that provides logical thinking and guidance to achieve informed decisions in healthcare practice.

FURTHER READING

Fletcher, R.H. and Fletcher, S.W. (2005) *Clinical Epidemiology: The Essentials*, 4th edn. Philadelphia: Lippincott, Williams and Wilkins.

Friis, R.H. and Sellers, T.A. (2004) *Epidemiology for Public Health Practice*, 3rd edn. Boston: Jones and Bartlett.

8 Public Health and Population Dynamics

Mzwandile (Andi) Mabhala and Walid El Ansari

DEFINITION

Demography is defined as the study of the size, structure, dispersement and development of human populations in order to establish reliable statistics on such factors as birth and death rates, marriages and divorces, life expectancy, and migration (Earle et al., 2007). It has been recognised that the understanding of the size, structure, past and future development of a population is fundamental to an understanding of its health. Therefore this understanding is regarded as a prerequisite for making the forecasts about future population size and structure which should underpin healthcare planning (Grundy, 2004). Demography is premised on the study of information that is gathered from population census or vital statistic records.

KEY POINTS

- Understanding demography is a prerequisite for making forecasts about future population size and structure which should underpin healthcare planning.
- Life expectancy is an important parameter in defining the size of a population because for a given birth rate the number of people is proportional to it.
- In terms of overall world population growth, migration will not affect global population change.
- High level and trends of fertility do not necessarily mean fast population growth.

DISCUSSION

Population dynamics

The notion of population growth and the effect it will have on the health of the population, and on the economy and the environment has been a preoccupation of health professionals, environmentalists and politicians. However, as we can see from the above scenario, a comprehensive view of all the dimensions of population change has been missing in every discussion. It would seem that a balanced and comprehensive analysis of the population dynamics (factors that affect the size, growth and structure of populations, as well as the interactions of these factors) is one that takes into consideration the data on the population 'stock' and on 'flow' in and out – births, migration and deaths (Earle et al., 2007).

Mechanisms that influence the size of a population

It has been established that the three mechanisms that control the size of a population are life expectancy at various ages, the fertility rate and migration (Grundy, 2004; US Census Bureau, 2004). However, Grundy further argues that of the three demographic determinants of population size, fertility is nearly always of much greater importance to both mortality and migration.

Population growth and fertility

The logical way of looking at population growth is to view it as a function of the balance between fertility and mortality and the extent of net migration. In other words, if the number of births is greater than the number of deaths, the size of the globe's population will grow.

In many developing countries the levels and the trends of fertility, if considered separately from the trends and level of mortality, could give a false impression that the population is growing quickly; but if one looks at these two indicators together one begins to notice that a large number of children disappear before their fifth birthday; a further rapid decrease can be observed between the ages of 20 and 45, and octogenarians are almost absent.

This impression of fast growth has led policy-makers, family planning programme managers and demographers to watch it avidly, to determine whether the growth is consistent with the notion of sustainable development. On the other hand, in developed countries where fertility is now at historic lows, these same vital statistics are examined for signs of a rise in fertility to the replacement levels needed to prevent future decline in population size (Bongaarts and Griffith, 1998).

Migration

Following years of studying the global population trends, the U.S. Census Bureau (2004) reached the conclusion that migration is not of sufficient magnitude to have a major impact on national population growth. This is contrary to the popular political view as observed in the above scenario. It has been established that every person who leaves one country must enter another, so net world migration will always equal zero. However, if net migration – that is, the difference between the numbers of people entering and leaving an area – is positive, the size of the population will grow, or else remain constant. According to the U.S. Census Bureau, in relative terms, the countries where net migration had the most impact on population size in the year 2000 (whether positive or negative) were either island nations or nations with recent experience of military conflict. For the majority of larger countries, however, the relative effect of net migration was small to moderate (U.S. Census

Bureau, 2004). However, the Office for National Statistics (2006) argues that migration – international migration in particular – is concentrated in the young adult years, therefore there is a significant second generation effect on births, with the number of women migrants increasing in childbearing age. This view is shared by Grundy (2004), who postulates that because international migrants are generally young and in good health, and often move from relatively high fertility populations to low fertility populations, they may serve to rejuvenate the host population and, at least initially, have higher fertility and lower mortality.

Life expectancy and population growth

Recently, life expectancy has been recognised as an important parameter in defining the size of a population because for a given birth rate the number of people is proportional to it (Marchette et al., 2007). In terms of population growth it has been observed that whilst one of the major successes of public health in the twentieth century has been reducing infant mortality, there has been an increase in life expectancy as the same time (Donaldson and Donaldson, 2003; Marchette et al., 2007). The gain in life expectancy has been occurring concurrently with the decrease in fertility, which has somewhat masked the effect of fertility. There has been concern, however, that the effect of increasing life expectancy on populations, which for a while has masked the decrease in fertility in some rich countries, will disappear (Marchette et al., 2007).

CASE STUDY

On Sunday 14 October 2007, on a TV political programme, a local MP expressed concern about the number of immigrants coming into the United Kingdom (UK). He quoted that in 2006 the UK received 600,000 immigrants, 300,000 from European Union (EU) countries and 300,000 from non-EU countries. He accepts that there is nothing that the UK can do about the EU immigrants but something needs to be done about the immigrants from outside EU countries, otherwise the UK economy will not be able to cope with the population increase. The main parts of the economy that he maintains will particularly struggle with the increasing demands are: schools, healthcare services, housing and employment.

CONCLUSION

The growth of the world population is at an all-time high in absolute numbers. While it took 123 years for the world population to double from 1 billion to 2 billion, succeeding increments of 1 billion took 33 years, 14 years and 13 years. Although the average woman worldwide is giving birth to fewer children than ever before, such increases have implications for the ultimate size and regional distribution of the world population and for prospects for sustainable development.

Demographic changes are important for industry and business, as well as for government planning in education, housing, welfare, transport and taxation. For example, in relation to the challenges of population ageing, the forecast rise in the number of people aged 75+ over the next 20 years will increase demand for accommodation for the elderly. Similarly, in relation to social/policy issues and the consequences of changes in family circumstances on the availability of informal sources of care and for older people's social participation, the fact that there are fewer children will put pressure on informal care and pensions costs for older populations. Likewise, advertising uses demographic information, where providers of services and goods need such information to reach the greatest number of possible clients in their target audience.

The demographic characteristics of a population could be affected by its history and biology, and are intertwined with its public health planning, economics and business decisions. Demography has wide socio-political implications as well as repercussions in relation to ethnicity, religion and nationalism. Further, if sustainable consumption and production are to be maintained, we will need to consider the population of working age as well as the proportion of dependants in a population: the non-working young and non-working old. Major shifts in a nation's changing age structures have broad socio-cultural consequences. Likewise, fertility might be affected by religion (high fertility in very religious populations); social customs (stigma as regards contraception); and education (a higher education level is associated with lower numbers of children). Moreover, due to both the unprecedented number of people alive and the ease of travel, the global movement of people has continued on the largest scale in history. Migration results in the numbers and distribution of people within a region being changed. It also stretches the limits of urban housing development and when it is inadequate for the influx of migrants, then ghettos/shanty towns are formed, and urban areas in developing regions contain more males.

According to the demographic transition theory, as living standards rise and health conditions improve, mortality rates should decline, followed by a decline in fertility rates some time later. But different societies experience the demographic transition at different rates. Hence, data gathered and studied for a demographic understanding of a population are determined by the groups or organisations who sourced the information. This could include whether the focus is on overall population and factors that alter it as a whole (births, deaths, migrations), or changes in its composition (sex, age, marital status, language, religion, race/ethnic grouping, family unit structure, housing, education, income, etc.). Such data could be used to forecast demand for facilities and services, and could be used by state organisations or other voluntary agencies to anticipate growth or decline and to plan and develop programmes and community resources.

FURTHER READING

Grundy, E. (2004) *Demography and Public Health*. Oxford: Oxford University Press.
Office for National Statistics (2006) *Population Trends*. London: Office for National Statistics.

9 Population Surveillance

Hamed A. Adetunji

DEFINITION

According to the definition of the Centers for Disease Control and Prevention (2001), public health surveillance is 'the ongoing, systematic collection, analysis, interpretation, and dissemination of data regarding a health-related event for use in public health action to reduce morbidity and mortality and to improve health'. Through these processes, infectious diseases or other health-related issues that can be potential threats to the health of populations can be identified and tracked before such threats become reality. To be meaningful, data collected on a continuous basis need to be carefully collated, analysed and interpreted, and the information disseminated promptly to those who require it for appropriate action to be taken. In the UK, the Health Protection Agency (HPA) is responsible for the communicable diseases surveillance while the Centers for Disease Control (CDC) does the same in the USA.

KEY POINTS

- To be meaningful, data collected on a continuous basis need to be collated, analysed, interpreted and disseminated.
- The final report of surveillance should be disseminated to all levels of public health practice.
- Public health surveillance system is essential for immediate and long-term public health action.
- Public health surveillance system is essential for disease prevention and control.
- Dissemination of information to all parties concerned with the data.
- Use the information for population health action.
- To reduce morbidity, mortality, and improve health.
- To make meaningful decisions for prevention and control of such diseases or other health threats.

DISCUSSION

Aims of surveillance

Surveillance is a central feature of epidemiology (see chapter 7). It is used for disease control and prevention. The main aims of public health surveillance include the following:

- *Primary prevention*: where risk factor(s) can be identified in order to prevent a disease's occurrence, as in the case of smoking and lung cancer;
- *Secondary prevention*: where disease is detected at the earliest stage so as to allow effective treatment/intervention at this stage when the survival rate can be improved, as in the case of using mammography to detect possible breast cancer;

- *Tertiary prevention*: where the risk factors are examined so as to put in place appropriate intervention that can alter the progression of adverse effect, as in the case of changing lifestyle or diet in relation to heart disease.

Principles of public health surveillance programmes

The following principles have been suggested as key for an effective surveillance system (Pencheon et al., 2006):

- Formulate clear objectives and design surveillance relevant to meeting the objectives.
- Collect exact data required to address only the stated objectives.
- Perform the direct measures of the condition under surveillance first followed by indirect measure.
- Maintain good personal relationships with all concerned.
- Show the importance of data collected to all parties involved in the collection.
- Give correct guidance and support to all parties involved in data collection when required.
- Predict barriers that would hinder a swift reporting system and guard against these arising.
- Provide routine analysis and interpretation of data by time, place and person.
- Make the analysis and interpretation of data part of the system down the line of the organisational structure.
- Disseminate the importance of the surveillance in epidemiology and in relation to public health practice.

Criteria for disease surveillance

The following criteria need to be fulfilled before disease surveillance begins:

- The disease must have a high public health impact.
- The disease must have a significant potential to become epidemic.
- There must be a significant public health action taken or that can be taken.
- The surveillance must be feasible.

The main sources of surveillance data are:

• Notifiable diseases – some diseases, as soon as symptoms are noticed or diagnosed by the attending doctor, must be reported to the appropriate office of communicable disease control.
• Laboratory reports – if a doctor sends a sample from a patient for testing, the laboratory can confirm what micro-organism (if any) is making the person sick.
• Clinician reporting – in some diseases of significance to public health, clinicians are required to report certain information so that appropriate public health action may be taken (see www.hpa.org.uk).

Data to be used in surveillance can also come from sources such as admission registers of hospitals, laboratory reports, cancer registries, population surveys, work/school sickness absence reports, cause of death reports and morbidity and mortality reports. Sources may also include the reports of epidemic inquiries, reports of inquiries into individual cases, and vaccination or population immunity level data. In England for example, the Office of National Statistics collects surveillance data continuously so that it can monitor whether an epidemic is occurring.

Dissemination of surveillance information

The final report of surveillance should be disseminated to all parties that need to know, especially at all levels of public health – local, regional, national and international. Knowledge of the patterns of disease occurrence in a particular local or regional setting will enable physicians to make appropriate diagnoses, leading to prompt and effective treatment. This will prevent the spread which is a crucial control measure. It also gives health services planners accurate information on which to base appropriate health policies. These can be used by public health professionals to commission appropriate health intervention to prevent and control the disease burden in the locality concerned and to prevent epidemics (Benenson, 1995).

How useful is surveillance information?

Data disseminated by a public health surveillance system can be used for immediate public health action. For example, it can be used to: provide knowledge of the natural history of a disease, to detect changes in the trends or distribution of the disease so that further investigative or control measures can be commenced; evaluate the trend of disease or health-related events; monitor continuously the occurrence and spread of disease that may be suitable for control. Other purposes include prioritising the allocation of resources for health intervention, to justify the need to carry out exploratory research and to identify research gaps (Pencheon et al., 2006).

How is surveillance designed?

- Define the problem.
- Identify opportunities for prevention and control.
- Set objectives.
- Specify requirements to meet the set objectives.
- Design the programme (highlighting case definition, data requirement, sources of data).
- Translate the designed information into action.
- Evaluate the programme.

CASE STUDY

Mr Patterson works in a local council as an information officer. One morning, while going through reports of the morbidity and mortality in the locality he noticed that there were 200 cases of heart attack deaths in his community in the year that had just ended. He alerted his superior officer, who also saw the need to do something. This figure appeared too high, according to their perception. The attention of the Primary Healthcare Trust was called to this, and the appropriate officer in the public health team – Dr David, a public health consultant – was asked to interpret the figure. He realised that the information in the report on its own was not enough to conclude that there had been an epidemic of heart attacks in the area. He tried to compare it with the previous year but this was not a good indication, in that some information that would enable the real pattern to be evaluated was missing. He therefore decided to set up a surveillance programme to evaluate the patterns of heart attack from then on, by size, age and sex of the population affected. The programme was carried out continuously for three years. Patterns were therefore monitored from the previous year to the new three-year data. It was discovered that the rate noticed at the beginning was actually the start of a decline in deaths due to heart attack in the community. Also, the rates compared favourably with other communities and there was no need to change the current interventions as they seemed to be working. There was no need to panic. Wrong messages could have been sent if this surveillance programme had not been set up.

FURTHER READING

Friis, R.H. and Sellers, T.A. (2004) *Epidemiology for Public Health Practice*, 3rd edn. Boston: Jones and Bartlett.

Benenson, A.S. (1995) *Control of Communicable Diseases Manual*, 16th edn. Washington, DC: American Public Health Association.

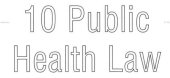

10 Public Health Law

Nicholas Fulton Phin

DEFINITION

Legislation aimed at preventing disease, prolonging life and promoting health, either directly or indirectly, is prolific and diverse, tackling issues as varied as smoking in public places, building and planning regulations, the wearing of seat belts and health and safety at work. Given this diversity of legislation, this chapter will deal with public health legislation as it relates to the prevention, surveillance and control of infectious diseases.

Rarely used legislation – section 47 of the National Assistance Act 1948 and the National Assistance (Amendment) Act 1951, permitting local authorities to remove an individual from their home to a place of safety – is not considered here. This legislation is considered by many to be inconsistent with the European Convention of Human Rights.

KEY POINTS

- The Public Health (Control of Disease) Act 1984 provides the legal framework to monitor and control infectious diseases.
- A new Health and Social Care Bill is expected in 2009.
- The Health and Social Care Bill will allow greater legal flexibility in the way infectious diseases are monitored and controlled and will extend the provisions of the Act to include infection or contamination (including radiation) which may present significant harm to health.

DISCUSSION

The Public Health (Control of Disease) Act 1984 represents the consolidation of over 130 years of legislation relating to infectious diseases and it is the primary legislation covering infectious diseases. The provisions of this Act and the Public Health (Infectious Disease) Regulations 1988 provide the current legal framework within which infectious diseases are monitored and controlled. It is therefore important to consult both of these pieces of legislation when considering any issues related to public health law.

The Public Health Act 1984 consists of six sections covering administrative and jurisdiction matters, the execution of the Act and a description, and the scope, of the powers available to monitor and control disease. Most duties and powers described within the Act and the Regulations are the responsibility of local authorities; however, the exercising of specific powers, for example the notification of diseases, is often delegated to named individuals, usually a consultant in communicable disease control (CCDC).

The key sections of the 1984 Act are in Part II and Part III where the powers available for the control of disease are described. Essentially the powers within the Act are divided into;

- surveillance – sections 10–18, 22, 39;
- investigation – sections 35–36, 40;
- controlling transmission – sections 19–21, 23–34, 37, 38, 41–45.

Surveillance

Section 11 of the 1984 Act is the most significant as this places a legal obligation on a registered medical practitioner (not the laboratory or anyone else) to notify the local authority if he becomes aware, or suspects, that a patient he is attending is suffering from a notifiable disease (listed in the 1988 Regulations) or from food poisoning. Notification takes the form of a certificate sent to the proper officer (usually the CCDC) containing certain prescribed personal information for which the medical practitioner receives a payment. Failure to comply with this duty can result in prosecution.

Investigation

Section 35 of the 1984 Act allows, on application to a justice of the peace, for an order requiring the examination of a person where there is reason to believe that the person may be suffering from a notifiable disease. Such an examination could include X-rays or any other bacteriological tests felt necessary. Sections 36 and 40 make reference to the examination of people or groups of people staying in a common lodging house where a notifiable disease is suspected.

Controlling transmission

A variety of powers exist for the control of transmission; sections 21 and 23 excluding children from school and places of entertainment; section 25 and 31, ordering the disinfection of library books and premises and finally sections 37 and 38 where, on application to a justice of the peace, it is possible to remove a person to hospital and to detain them there if they are suspected to be suffering from a notifiable disease.

The Public Health (Infectious Disease) Regulations 1988, in addition to listing the notifiable diseases and the provisions of the 1984 Act that apply to each, also provides for additional measures that can be instituted to control disease. Of particular interest is section 10 of the Regulations which allows the proper officer of a district where a case of a notifiable disease occurs to arrange (through the Primary Care Trust) the vaccination or immunisation, without charge, of any person in her district who has come or may have come or may come into contact with the infection.

Recent changes to the International Health Regulations approved by the Health Assembly of the World Health Organization (WHO) in 2005, and to which the UK is a signatory, have necessitated a review of the Public Health (Control of Disease) Act 1984. This is considered by many to be long overdue since the relevance of certain provisions of the

Act, consolidated over many years, are of questionable application in modern society, for example, section 25 relating to the disinfection of library books. In addition, the current list of notifiable diseases has failed to keep pace with the new emerging diseases such as SARS and E Coli O157.

The review undertaken and consulted on in 2007 recommended a number of changes (HPA, 2007), most of which have been incorporated into the Health and Social Care Bill which is expected to become law in the UK later in 2008. These include:

- changes to international travel regulations, including allowing regulations to be made covering the detention, examination and decontamination of conveyances, the examination, isolation, quarantine and decontamination of people and detention, examination and decontamination of things;
- changes to domestic regulations, include expanding the Act to allow the inclusion of any infection or contamination (including radiation) which presents or could present significant harm to human health; powers to allow a justice of the peace to order health measures in relation to persons, e.g. submit to medical examination, isolation or quarantine and decontamination; powers to allow a justice of the peace to order health measures in relation to things, e.g. destruction or decontamination.

The case study below attempts to demonstrate how the 1984 Act might be applied when dealing with a notifiable disease.

CASE STUDY

Mrs Smith is a nursery nurse who visited her general practitioner (GP) because of weight loss, night sweats and a persistent productive cough. She had visited South Africa to care for a sick relative in the three months prior to her symptoms. The GP suspected pulmonary tuberculosis and informed her that she needed further investigation and that he would be notifying the local Health Protection Unit of her possible diagnosis. She became angry, refused to be investigated and threatened to report the doctor to the General Medical Council if he breached her right to privacy. When advised to stay off work, she insisted that there was nothing wrong with her and she could not afford to stay off work or keep her children out of school. The head teacher of the school when approached for details of the children in the classes that Mrs Smith taught refused, under the Data Protection Act, to supply the CCDC with any information.

Tuberculosis is a notifiable disease and, under section 11 of the Public Health Act 1984, her GP is under a legal obligation to notify the proper officer (often the CCDC) of the local authority if he believes that any of his patients may be suffering from tuberculosis, whether open pulmonary TB or a closed lesion affecting any other tissue. The right to privacy described in the Human Rights Act would not apply since public health measures such as this are a matter of public interest and override anyone's right to privacy.

If the patient could not be persuaded to have any investigations, then the CCDC could make an application under section 35 of the 1984 Act to a justice of the peace for an order requiring the patient to be examined by a nominated medical practitioner and undergo X-ray and/or bacteriological investigations. Failure to submit to this would lead to further legal action.

In relation to her work, any person who, knowing they may be suffering from a notifiable disease, carries on working when the risk of spreading infection cannot be excluded, can be prosecuted under section 19 of the 1984 Act.

Until the children of the patient have been investigated and declared free of the infection, under section 21 of the 1984 Act, it would be possible to exclude them from school until the proper officer was satisfied they were free of infection.

The head teacher's refusal to give information on his pupils is misguided; the Data Protection Act would not apply in this instance given the overriding public interest issue. However, should it be necessary, section 22 of the 1984 Act could be used to require the head teacher to provide a list of pupils within a specified department, within a reasonable fixed time. Failure to do so could result in prosecution.

Mrs Smith eventually agrees to be examined but despite the diagnosis of open pulmonary tuberculosis, declines treatment and insists on attending various social events. Given the high prevalence of multi-drug-resistant tuberculosis in South Africa, where it is thought likely that she acquired the infection, it is considered imperative that treatment is started as soon as possible. In this situation the CCDC could apply to a justice of the peace using section 37 for an order requiring her removal to hospital and an application under section 38 for her detention there. It is important to note that although the patient can be taken to hospital and detained there, the Public Health Act 1984 does not have the power to require patients to undergo treatment.

CONCLUSION

However, until the enactment of the new legislation and the creation of the various new regulations that will flow from it, the current Public Health (Control of Disease) Act 1984 and the Public Health (Infectious Disease) Regulations 1988 will still provide the legal authority for the surveillance, prevention and management of infectious disease in England and Wales.

FURTHER READING

Detels, R., McEwen, J., Beaglehole, R. and Tanaka, H. (2002) *Oxford Textbook of Public Health*, 4th edn. Oxford: Oxford University Press.

11 Leadership Development for Public Health Practitioners

Frances Wilson and Kim Greening

Delivering the public health agenda requires well developed leadership skills, subject expertise and a comprehensive knowledge of public health and its application.

DEFINITION

Leaders can be defined as:

> People who make things happen in ways that command the confidence of local staff. They are people who lead teams, people who lead service networks, people who lead partnerships, and people who lead organisations. (King's Fund, 2004b)

This definition clearly suggests that leadership occurs at all levels within an organisation. In terms of the qualities that are central to leadership at any level England's Chief Medical Officer (DH, 2001a) proposes that:

> A leader must be able to inspire and be seen to have integrity. These qualities will develop more easily by someone who works in a team, who learns effectively and who communicates and explains policy. A leader who sees quickly to the heart of a problem will be able to position himself or herself and be able to gauge situations correctly.

The National Health Service (NHS) vision for leadership development is directly linked with the modernisation agenda and the need for change, innovation and improvement at all levels in the organisation (DH, 2000b).

Many other definitions of leaders and leadership exist, but which of these is appropriate will depend on the local public health agreements and impetus for change such as the impact of national policies, partnership and inter-agency working arrangements (Goodwin cited in Griffiths and Hunter, 2007).

KEY POINTS

- The drivers for leadership development.
- Acquiring leadership skills.
- The Leadership Awareness model.
- Related academic theory.

DISCUSSION

The policy documents summarised in Box 11.1 contain some of the key drivers for leadership development amongst health professionals in the last decade. The focus of leadership has been strengthened and developed with the aim of improving patient services by leading change and influencing commissioning at corporate level. To effect the public health agenda in the twenty-first century NHS education and training in leadership are key to success.

Box 11.1 *A summary of policy documents driving leadership development*

Making a Difference (DH, 1999) – The strategy for nursing emphasised strengthening nursing leadership to achieve the government's modernisation programme. Nurses, midwives and health visitors need enhanced leadership skills to boost leadership and management across the NHS.

NHS Plan (DH, 2000b) – The NHS Leadership Centre was established in 2001 to promote leadership development closely linked to the Modernisation Agency's work to deliver improved patient services across all professional levels.

Liberating the Talents (DH, 2002) – This provides a new framework for nursing in primary care to promote leadership development for those in new specialist and advanced practitioner roles through e.g. LEO, RCN and the Nursing Leadership Centre programmes. More nurses will lead and deliver public health programmes, the concept of corporate leadership is introduced, the potential of all practitioners to be leaders is highlighted and there is an emphasis on transformational leadership style.

Choosing Health (DH, 2004b) – Here there is a new emphasis on delivering health improvements through promotion of leadership and public health in health and social care – this may be through facilitating community leadership, strategic partnerships, supporting the development of effective specialist public health practice and leadership skills.

Our Health Our Care Our Say (DH, 2006e) – Strong effective leadership is needed at PCT level to enhance commissioning and promote co-termination between healthcare services and local government.

Our NHS, Our Future (DH, 2007e) – This suggests leadership is built into formal and informal education and training for all professional groups, identifies role models, and encourages healthcare professionals to take up leadership roles as part of their career path.

How public health practitioners acquire leadership skills varies. Practitioners may attend full or part time courses to acquire the knowledge, skills and competencies to become a specialist community public health nurse (NMC, 2004) or become a Master in Public Health

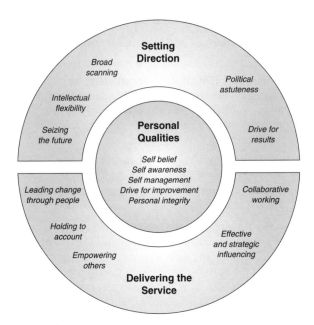

Figure 11.1   *The NHS Leadership Qualities Framework (NHS Leadership Centre 2001)*

(MPH). Such knowledge, skills and competencies will be mapped into educational programmes to ensure provenance, quality and fitness for purpose.

Alternatively, public sector managerial and business degrees incorporate leadership content designed to be applied at board level within a Primary Care Trust or in commissioning roles.

More specifically, the NHS Leadership Centre was launched in 2001. The centre emerged from the vision of the NHS Plan (DH, 2000b) to enable those in senior leadership positions and aspiring leaders to analyse and develop their skills using the NHS Leadership Qualities Framework (LQF) (Figure 11.1). It was developed through studying the qualities of successful leaders and distilling those qualities into an assessment tool (NHS Leadership Centre, 2001).

The framework is organised into three sections designed to assess personal qualities, setting direction and delivering the service. Knowing one's self is central to being a successful leader, setting a vision for the future and leading transformational change through people. When designing a leadership programme for public health and community practitioners, many organisations utilise LQF guidelines (NHS Leadership centre, 2004) or base programmes on them.

Successful leadership development is provided by universities, NHS Trusts, the King's Fund, Royal College of Nursing, Royal College of Midwives and other organisations. Ultimately, the goals of all programme participants should be to impact positively on patient care, empower others, influence public health policy and effect organisational change.

'Leading Empowered Organisations' (LEO) and 'Leadership at the Point of Care' programmes are examples designed to support the practical application of such skills by practitioners at team leader and ward manager levels (King's Fund, 2004b; Hancock and Campbell, 2006).

More recently a UK Career Framework for Public Health has been developed. The framework is described as coherent and flexible and the initiative itself as 'the first time public health competences, underpinning knowledge, training and qualification routes, registration requirements and a database of job descriptions across nine career levels are being brought together in a user friendly format' (Public Health Resource Unit, 2007).

This exciting development has a leadership element as a core theme entitled 'Leadership and collaborative working for health'. This competency may be applied throughout an organisation, for example at senior strategic level to directors of public health, public health doctors and consultant practitioners; at organisational level to advanced and specialist practitioners, team leaders, public health nurses (health visitors, school nurses and occupational health nurses), district nurses and those working in supporting roles such as assistant and associate practitioners.

Using leadership skills to improve public health requires practitioners to work in partnership with other workers, with communities and across organisational boundaries. Additionally the following skills are considered essential: leading and managing teams; building alliances; developing capacity and capability; working in partnership with other practitioners and agencies, and using the media effectively to improve health and wellbeing.

CASE STUDY – USING THE LEADERSHIP AWARENESS MODEL

The framework shown in Figure 11.2 is advanced as an inter-professional educational model incorporating the essential elements required for successful leadership development.

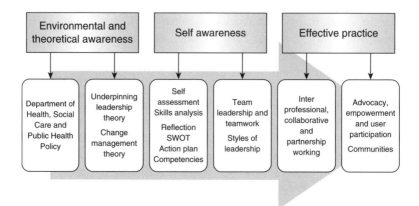

Figure 11.2 *Leadership Awareness Model*

The model is used to underpin the leadership curriculum in the Faculty of Health and Social Care, University of Chester for public health practitioners and other health professionals. It mirrors the LQF in that its central focus is on the development of self-awareness with regard to leadership styles, strengths and weaknesses.

Students embark on a journey of self-discovery by viewing their own leadership (past, present and future) from a range of perspectives. Self-assessment tools such as Myers-Briggs type indicators and Belbin's Team roles (Belbin, 1993) are used to aid self-analysis in addition to one or two substantial reflective pieces of writing. By using two or three tools and triangulating the results, practitioners identify areas for personal development. This can be followed through using a SWOT analysis and action plans, incorporating goals and practical challenges, to enhance strengths or to develop confidence in acquiring new skills.

Due to the nature of the leadership development – it is about personal development and can at times be painful for the participants – an action learning approach is adopted.

Action Learning is based on the relationship between reflection and action ... where the focus is on the issues and problems that individuals bring and planning future action with the structured attention and support of the group. (Fry et al., 2002)

key concepts in public health

At every stage throughout the self-assessment the student's analysis is informed by relevant leadership theory: transformational leadership; team building; change management; systems thinking. Students appreciate that a transformational style is required to communicate a vision, inspire and motivate individuals or for a team to innovate and introduce change in the workplace. If specific tasks are to be undertaken or directed then a transactional style may be more appropriate. They also learn that a good leader will be able to adapt or switch their style according to circumstances utilising a situational leadership approach. Dispersed or emergent leadership is another model that is promoted and aligns with the proposal for corporate leadership (DH, 2002) in that all individuals in an organisation have the potential to be leaders given the right circumstances, education and support (Bolden et al., 2003; DH, 2007b).

The Improvement Leaders' Guides (NHS Institute for Innovation and Improvement, 2005) provide an excellent resource; they contain many practical ideas and examples that help students apply theory to their own workplace situation. Listening to 'patient stories' is a powerful tool used to explore advocacy, empowerment, partnership working and community engagement in terms of understanding the patient experience and ultimately improving public health.

CONCLUSION

Leadership development in the NHS is driven by public health and the health and social care agenda. The focus of leadership activity is to lead an educated, skilled workforce capable of implementing change in public health practice and service delivery and together empower people and communities to achieve a healthy lifestyle balance.

FURTHER READING

Skills for Health (2007) *Multidisciplinary/multi-agency/multi-professional public health skills and career framework – Consultation version.* Oxford: NHS Public Health Resource Unit. Retrieved 28 March 2008, from http://www.phru.nhs.uk
NHS Institute for Innovation and Improvement – (2005) *Leadership qualities framework.* Retrieved 28 March 2008, from http://www.nhsleadershipqualities.nhs.uk/

development leadership

12 Social Marketing

Allison Thorpe, Rowena Merritt, Clive Blair-Stevens and Jeff French

DEFINITION

Social marketing is a customer-centred behavioural intervention approach that can be used to help achieve and sustain different behaviour over time. In the 1970s when it was coined as a term it was largely seen as the use of commercial marketing methods for social good. However, since then it has become a much more mature and integrative discipline. It is sometimes referred to as having 'two parents': the 'social parent', which draws from the range of social and behavioural sciences, and the 'marketing parent'.

Debate and discussion within the wider public health and health improvement fields, and in social marketing in particular, has increasingly moved beyond a limited individual focus to consider the wider determinants of health and the potential for harnessing marketing approaches to secure social benefits.

In formal terms social marketing has been defined as *'the systematic application of marketing, alongside other concepts and techniques, to achieve specific behavioural goals, for a social good'* (French and Blair-Stevens, 2006). This definition highlights the systematic nature of social marketing, while also emphasising its behavioural focus and its primary concern with a 'social good'. The main differences between commercial and social marketing are compared in Table 12.1.

KEY POINTS

- Social marketing is an integrative approach drawing on social sciences and marketing.
- It is driven by a strong customer orientation, seeking to develop a deep understanding and insight into what influences, moves and motivates people.

Table 12.1 *A comparison of commercial sector marketing and social marketing*

	Commercial marketing	Social marketing
Product	The marketing process is used to selling of goods and services and promote 'brand value'	The marketing process is used to promote and sustain positive behaviour for a social good
Primary aim	Financial gain and share-holder value	Social benefits for individuals and communities
Competition	Other companies selling goods or services	Any factors that undermine the sustaining of the desired behaviour

Source: National Social Marketing Centre (NSMC) (2007). Adapted from Kotler et al. (2002).

- Its overriding concern is with achieving and sustaining specific behaviour.
- It does not focus on individuals in isolation, but seeks to understand them in their wider social and environmental context.
- Social marketing techniques are not restricted to the health field, but are increasingly used across a range of social policy areas.

DISCUSSION

Social marketing has not traditionally been widely integrated into preventative or behavioural intervention approaches in the UK, although it has been more widely used in Canada, the USA, New Zealand and Australia. Recently there has been a growing cross-government appreciation of its potential to help improve the impact and effectiveness of behavioural interventions in the UK which is reflected in an increased profile and integration into policy and practice, with the Department of Health being a particular champion of the approach.

The 'It's our health!' independent review report, commissioned by the Department of Health, has been particularly influential. This affirmed the potential of social marketing and provided a set of practical recommendations to help build capacity and skills and promote its wider use and integration at national and local levels.

Key features – the national benchmark criteria

With the wider integration of social marketing into national policy and practice there has been a growing concern that existing methods may simply be re-badged as 'social marketing' and lead to a distorted view of what social marketing really involves. In order to tackle this issue and to help build a wider consistency of approach a set of national benchmark criteria were developed and published (French and Blair-Stevens, 2006). These consist of eight key criteria which characterise social marketing approaches (see Table 12.2).

A simple device for helping to highlight the key features of social marketing, is the social marketing 'customer triangle' (see Figure 12.1).

Successful social marketing programmes reflect a logical planning process, which can be used at both individual and strategic policy development levels. The Total Process Planning model (Figure 12.2) is a simple conceptualisation of the process, which in practice can be challenging to action. The emphasis placed on the front end 'scoping stage' of the model, and its role in establishing clear actionable and measurable behaviour goals to ensure focused development across the rest of the process is a key determinant of success.

CASE STUDY

Successful social marketing approaches ensure that all intervention methods and approaches incorporated can be tracked back and measured in terms of their influence on people's actual behaviour, not just awareness of the message transmitted. The 'Truth' study provides a good illustration of how this works in practice. Following successful litigation against the tobacco companies, the State of Florida decided to invest the realised funds in an upstream health promotion intervention, which demonstrated considerable success in reducing underage smoking rates. The case study demonstrates the eight national benchmark characteristics of social marketing interventions (see Table 12.2).

Over the last five to ten years, the evidence base on social marketing has continued to develop, and increasingly demonstrates its potential for improving the impact and effectiveness of interventions. It has been successfully applied to various health campaigns with a diversity of aims, including reducing teenage smoking rates and pregnancies, promoting safe gun storage, and preventing youth suicide (Kotler et al., 2002).

Table 12.2 *Social marketing National Benchmark Criteria*

Customer Orientation	Focuses on the 'customer in the round'. Developing a robust understanding of the audience based on good market and consumer research, combining data from different sources
Behaviour	Clear focus on behaviour based on a strong behavioural analysis, with development of specific behaviour goals
Theory	Behavioural theory-based and informed. Drawing on an integrated theory framework
Insight	Based on developing a deeper 'insight' approach – focusing on what 'moves and motivates' the consumer
Exchange	Incorporates an 'exchange' analysis. Understanding what the person has to give to get the benefits proposed
Competition	Incorporates a 'competition' analysis. Understanding what competes for the time and attention of the audience. Including both internal (psychological) and external competition
Segmentation	Uses a developed segmentation approach (not just targeting). Avoiding blanket approaches, tailoring work to people's different needs
Methods Mix	Identifies an appropriate 'mix of methods' rather than relying on a single approach (e.g. just communications). Used in strategic social marketing this can be described as the 'intervention mix'. Used in operational social marketing intervention the term 'marketing mix' may be used

Source: NSMC, 2006. Adapted from Andreasen (2002)

A new database of interventions, which will be regularly updated, can now be found at www.nsmcentre.org.uk.

Whilst much of the historical literature and examples of practice currently in the field of 'operational social marketing' focused on changing individual behaviour, a new 'strategic social marketing' approach is increasingly being developed. This approach seeks to look at ways that a

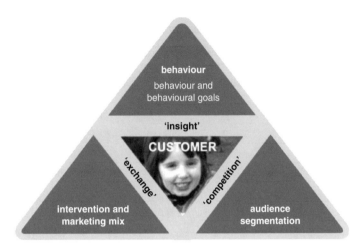

Figure 12.1 *Social marketing 'customer triangle'*

Source: NSMC, 2007

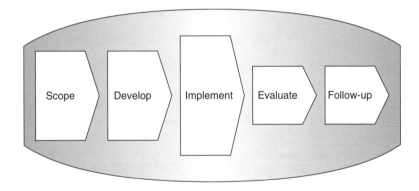

Figure 12.2 *The Total Process Planning model*

Source: NSMC, 2006

stronger customer understanding can inform policy development and strategic planning. This work is still at a relatively early stage, but the UK has taken a strong lead in this and the Department of Health and National Social Marketing Centre are actively working in this area.

Table 12.3 *Summary of 'truth' initiative against key benchmark criteria*

Benchmark criteria	'Truth' initiative
Customer orientation	Extensive research carried out to identify competition and possible levers
Behaviour	Reduction of uptake of smoking
Theory-base	Social benefits and norms. Community engagement and involvement. Life-stage development
Insight	Identified 'rebellion' and 'control' as key levers for youth (recognised that simply promoting 'being good and healthy' would be more likely to reinforce the negative behaviour)
Exchange	Promoted rebellion against control of tobacco industry
Competition	Understood nature of relationship with tobacco industry and specifically targeted this
Uses a segmentation approach	Focus was on young people with a particular emphasis on those most likely to take up smoking
Integrates a mix of methods	A wide range used including: community engagement and involvement strategies; social norm promotion; direct action interventions; media and PR engagement.

Source: NSMC (2007). Adapted from Kotler et al. (2002)

CONCLUSION

The potential of social marketing is increasingly being recognised with a growing evidence base that when applied systematically it has real potential to improve the impact and effectiveness of public health and other behavioural interventions. As an integrative discipline it is able to promote a much stronger customer-focused approach drawing on learning from both marketing and wider social sciences. The UK is still at a relatively early stage in its use and application but at policy, strategy and operational levels it is being used to support a wide range of social policy agendas and help address related behavioural challenges.

FURTHER READING

Hastings, G. (2007) *Social Marketing: The Potential.* London: Butterworth-Heinemann.

Kotler, P. and Lee, N. (2006) *Marketing in the Public Sector: A Roadmap for Improved Performance.* London: Financial Times/Prentice-Hall.

National Social Marketing Centre (2007) *Social Marketing: Big Pocket Guide.* London: NSMC.

13 Economics of Health

Hamed A. Adetunji

DEFINITION

Last (2007) defined economics as 'the branch of scholarly activity concerned with the production, consumption, transfer of goods, services and wealth and with the allocation of finite resources'. There are many branches of economics – microeconomics, macroeconomics and health economics. The concern of this chapter is health economics. Health economics is the discipline that enables health planners and practitioners to deal with the challenges brought about by scarcity of resources and the choice to arrive at in a logical manner so that accountabilities can be ensured. As Brambleby and Appleby cited in Pencheon et al. (2006) simply put it, health economics 'brings a systematic approach to the management of issues of scarcity and choice'. Public health practitioners and other healthcare workers will often face challenges when making decisions as to what programme of intervention needs to be put in place, how the programme will be justified in terms of value for money, and how its effectiveness will be measured. These and many other resource-related questions are what the health economics discipline answer in the day-to-day practice of public health and other healthcare.

KEY POINTS

- Health economics deals with production, consumption and allocation of resources to health programmes.
- It helps in the management of scarcity and choice issues.
- Health economics deals with effectiveness and efficiency in healthcare.

DISCUSSION

Application of health economics is a form of the economic evaluation of healthcare programmes. Economic evaluation has a similar definition to health economics, and at times is used synonymously. It is based on the concepts of scarcity of resources, opportunity cost and choices. Economic evaluation, according to Coyle and Davies (1996), 'addresses the question of whether an intervention or procedure is worth doing when compared with other possible uses of the same resources'. In fact, Drummond et al. (1997) simply defined economic evaluation as 'the comparative analysis of alternative courses of action in terms of both costs and the consequences'.

Why do public health practitioners and other healthcare professionals need health economics or economic evaluation? Knowledge of this discipline is important to them for many reasons: They are expected to make decisions about resource allocation; economic evaluation is a framework that simply makes a trade-off explicit; public health practitioners and other healthcare workers should be part of evaluation; Multidisciplinary evaluation is imperative, and they are going to be faced with an increasing managerial responsibilities.

Types of choice

Two types of choice in economics are the technical choice and the allocation choice. An example of technical choice is a question such as, 'What is the cheapest way of preventing the bird flu epidemic?' Allocation choice deals with questions such as, 'Should we invest in the smoking cessation project or in increasing the number of speed cameras on our roads?'

Efficiency in healthcare

Economic efficiency in healthcare services means making choices that maximise the benefit from the scarce resources available to the community. It involves appraisal of healthcare alternatives by calculating the amount by which the benefits derived exceed the costs expended. This economic evaluation involves calculation of both inputs and outputs, which are often referred to as costs and consequences (Drummond et al., 1997). The value of inputs and consequences of a programme are then compared with its alternatives.

There are four types of economic evaluation technique that are used in healthcare: cost-minimisation analysis, cost-effectiveness analysis, cost-benefit analysis and cost-utility analysis.

Cost-minimisation analysis   Cost-minimisation analysis searches for the lowest cost alternative. This technique is used when the two alternatives being considered produce identical consequences. For example, supposing one intends to find out which of two minor operations – day surgery of inguinal hernia or hospitalisation – will cost less. In both options the operations are successfully completed. The two result in the same outcome: the hernia is repaired. What is left is the difference in the cost of the two types of surgery, which is the cost per surgical procedure (Drummond et al., 1997).

Cost-effectiveness analysis   In cost-effectiveness analysis, two alternative programmes may have the same consequences (say prolonging life) but the cost of carrying out the two programmes may differ and so may their degree of success in achieving this common goal. Cost-effectiveness analysis is thus performed when the costs of alternative programmes are related to a single common outcome, which could be different in its degree of success. Cost-effectiveness analysis can be used to analyse alternatives that produce common consequences. For example, heart transplantation can be compared with compulsory seat belt wearing legislation since they produce similar effects 'in life years saved'. In the same way, hepatitis B immunisation programmes' consequences can be compared with kidney transplantation. Both perhaps have a common effect – cost per life year gained.

Cost-benefit analysis In the cost-effectiveness analysis explained above, consequences of alternatives might be identical. Most of the time this cannot be assessed. Also it may be difficult to have the outcomes common to the two alternatives reached to a single common effect. At times, the effects of alternatives under consideration may be multiple. Analyses which measure both the costs and the consequences of alternatives in dollars are called cost-benefit analyses.

Cost-benefit analyses provide information on the relative performance of programmes as well as on their 'absolute benefits'. In other words, the analysis provides a simulation of the value of resources that are used to perform each programme as well as the value of resources that might be saved or created by the programme.

Cost-utility analysis (CUA) The term 'utility' is used to show the preferences that individuals or society can have for a given set of health outcomes: that is, preferences that can be expressed on 'a given health state' or 'a profit of states over time'. Cost-utility analysis is a technique that uses utilities as a measure of the value of programme consequences. Its usefulness is especially due to the fact that it allows for 'quality of life' adjustments of a given set of programme consequences to be measured as well as providing a generic consequence measure for comparison including outcomes in alternative programmes.

None of these techniques can be regarded as superior to the others in that all depend on data and resources available.

The concept of costs

It is generally recommended that the programme being evaluated be looked at from the societal viewpoint even though, in the analysis, the implications for the donor agency or household budgets can be addressed as well. From the societal point of view, the cost elements to look at include: the costs of implementing the project, that is the cost incurred by the health sector (such as the labour costs); the cost incurred by the household (such as the time lost from work due to treatment or illness, the home care or the parent's time in taking the child to receive immunisation); and costs that may be incurred outside the health sector (for example, if the programme concerns children, school may incur certain costs).

economics of health

71

Measure of consequences

The major elements of consequences in economic evaluation include changes in functioning in relation to physical, social or emotional, usually termed health effects. In developed countries, analysts of economic evaluation of healthcare interventions are concerned mostly with evaluations of treatments of chronic conditions. In those conditions, treatment may not necessarily have much effect on the underlying conditions but will allow the patients some relief and provide improvements in the quality of lives. The indicators used to measure physical, social or emotional functioning can be specific to the disease concerned (for example, number of hepatitis B surface antigen 'HBsAg' cases prevented) or general, such as the number of deaths prevented.

CASE STUDY

Mr John is in charge of the immunisation programme in one of the Primary Care Trusts. He found that the immunisation uptake of a centre is doing better than another centre within his Trust. Before he jumped to the conclusion that the centre not doing so well should be cautioned he wanted to assess whether the resource inputs into the two centres were the same – he simply wanted to find out the cost per fully immunised child in the two centres. He then set out to do cost-effectiveness studies on immunisation. These can be divided into two categories according to the measure of effectiveness used: those that use the intermediate output of immunisation such as the number of fully immunised children, and those that use health impact such as the number of deaths prevented by immunisation. Mr John needs the former, in which the focus is on the internal efficacy of immunisation programmes whereby activities in different delivery areas are compared. With the help of a public health specialist in the trust, a simple study of cost-effectiveness in the two centres for cost incurred in fully immunising a child was carried out. The results showed the cost per fully immunised child in the centre that was doing well to be higher than the costs in the other centre: £4.39 as against £2.00. Rather than label the other centre ineffective and issue a caution, Mr John decided to look into the areas of adjustment to allocation of resources to make the other centre's immunisation uptake improve. The exercise helped Mr John to make an informed decision and avoided unnecessary action against the centre tagged as not doing well.

FURTHER READING

Jones, A. (2008) *Applied Econometrics for Health Economists*, 2nd edn. London: Office of Health Economics.
Mooney, G. (2003) *Economics, Medicine and Health Care*. Harlow: Pearson Education.

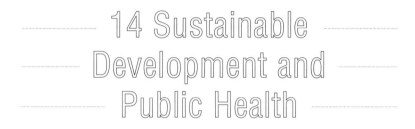

14 Sustainable Development and Public Health

Mzwandile (Andi) Mabhala and Peete Lesiamo

DEFINITION

The linkage between environment and development was globally recognized in 1980, when the International Union for the Conservation of Nature published the World Conservation Strategy and used the term 'sustainable development'. At that time sustainable development was primarily concerned with ecological sustainability, or the conservation of living resources, and little attention was directed to wider political, economic or social issues (Carter, 2001). Three non-governmental organisations – the International Union for the Conservation of Nature (IUCN), United Nations Environment Programme (UNEP) and World Wildlife Fund – met and defined 'sustainable development' as 'a socio-ecological process characterised by the fulfilment of human needs while maintaining the quality of the natural environment indefinitely'.

Since then the term 'sustainable development' has been popularised and given a broader political and social meaning by the World Commission on Environment and Development (WCED) in its WHO report entitled *Our Common Future* (WCED, 1987) commonly known as the Brundtland Report after the chair of the commission and former prime

sustainable development

73

minister of Norway, Gro Harlem Brundtland. The Brundtland Report coined what has become the universally used definition of sustainable development as 'development that meets the needs of the present without compromising the ability of future generations to meet their own needs'.

It is now recognised that sustainable development is about much more than environmental issues; it envelops policy issues such as creating stronger, healthy communities and economies, and promoting social cohesion, environmental and social concerns (WHO, 2000). Porritt for example defines sustainable development as: 'about improving the physical, social and personal quality of people's lives in a way that does not mess things up for the future generations' (Porritt, 2005).

KEY POINTS

- Sustainable development is about more than environmental issues; it envelops policy issues.
- The core objective of sustainable development is optimising human welfare.
- Reducing health inequalities, promoting and protecting health, prevention of disease and prolonging life are principles shared by public health and sustainable development.
- Sustainable development goals and targets are unlikely to be met unless efforts to reduce the gap between rich and poor are dramatically and rapidly scaled up.
- Poverty and environmental degradation are structured by uneven distribution of resources and uneven access to the opportunities for development technologies.

DISCUSSION

There are three interrelated elements shared by most definitions. First, the core objective of sustainable development is optimising human welfare. Welfare includes income and material consumption, along with education, health, equality of opportunity and human rights. The second objective is that all physical and economic activity should be compatible with the surrounding biosphere. This objective focuses on non-renewable resources, and emphasises that these should not be used at a rate that exceeds the rate at which they can be substituted by sustainable renewable resources. Thus, there should be no net degradation of the wide range of indispensable services provided by the natural environment. The third element is the equitable distribution of biospherically compatible improvements in human wellbeing, both today and tomorrow. Sustainability, in this context, implies both inter-generational and intra-generational equity. Human betterment on the part of any group should not come at the expense of other groups today or generations in the future.

The breadth of the definition and the objectives typifies the difficulty with practical implementation of sustainable development: if, for example, we want to demonstrate our commitment to sustainable development, what precisely are we expected to do? Despite universal acceptance of the definition of sustainable development as 'development that meets the needs of the present without compromising the ability of future generations to meet their own needs', agreement on what is meant by 'meets the need' remains a challenge. Jeffery (2006) argues that our perceptions of human needs depend to some extent on the society in which we live. Some would define 'needs' as the basic essentials of food, water and shelter. Others might include health provision and social security, while ultimately, there are the so-called 'needs' of many in the developed world for cars, washing machines, television, etc. This presents international policy-makers with a challenge in setting common international strategies for sustainable development.

National sustainable development strategies

The first call for the implementation of national sustainable development strategies (NSDS) was made at the UN Conference on Environment and Development (UNCED) in Rio in 1992. It was decided that countries should aim to complete strategies as soon as practicable, and if possible by 1994 (United Nations, 1992). Five years later, the 1997 Special Session of the UN General Assembly noted that there had been continued deterioration in the state of the global environment under the combined pressures of unsustainable production and consumption patterns, and population growth. This assessment led governments to reinforce their efforts by setting a new deadline of 2002 for 'the formulation and elaboration of national strategies for sustainable development' (United Nations, 1997).

The 2002 World Summit on Sustainable Development (WSSD) in Johannesburg called on all countries 'to make progress in the formulation and elaboration of national strategies for sustainable development and begin their implementation by 2005'. It encouraged 'relevant authorities at all levels to take sustainable development considerations into account in decision-making' (United Nations, 2002).

A study conducted by Swanson et al. (2004) for the International Institute for Sustainable Development (IISD), based on analysis of the national strategies of 19 countries, identified that few countries are acting truly strategically. The UK is amongst the 15 countries that developed 'comprehensive strategies'. The 2005 UK sustainable development strategy sets out five principles (Adshead et al., 2006):

- living within environmental limits;
- ensuring a strong, healthy and just society;
- achieving a sustainable economy;
- promoting good governance;
- using sound science responsibly.

Sustainable development, health and public health

The convergence of health and environment agendas was first made in the Rio Declaration on Environment and Development (United Nations, 1992). The first of 27 principles of sustainable development endorsed in Rio states that: 'Human beings are at the centre of concerns for sustainable development. They are entitled to a healthy and productive life in harmony with nature' (United Nations, 1992: 1).

The World Summit on Sustainable Development in Johannesburg (26 August to 4 September 2002) put health at the centre stage of sustainable development; it provided an opportunity to strengthen the role of health in sustainable development (United Nations, 2002). It made an explicit link between health, poverty, environment and sustainable development. It argued that the goals of sustainable development cannot be achieved when there is a high prevalence of debilitating illness and poverty, and that the health of a population cannot be maintained without a responsive health system and a healthy environment. Environmental degradation, mismanagement of natural resources, and unhealthy consumption patterns and lifestyles impact on health. Ill health, in turn, hampers poverty alleviation and economic development (United Nations, 2002).

WHO's Sustainable Development and Healthy Environments (SDE) programme identifies three unifying themes that underlie sustainable development and healthy environments (WHO, 2005):

- the promotion and protection of health as a human right;
- 'The importance of health in development goals such as the eradication of poverty and overcoming inequality';

- the recognition that human health needs to be protected from environmental hazards such as pollution, resource depletion and changes in ecosystems.

These themes are clearly resonant with the fundamental principles of public health: that is, reducing health inequalities, promoting and protecting health, preventing disease and prolonging life. The causes of poverty and environmental degradation are structured by uneven distribution of resources and uneven access to the opportunities for development – technologies, incentives, institutions and regulations which favour some over others (Masika and Joekes, 1997). Professor Buch began his talk at the 2002 WSSD by emphasising that sustainable development goals and targets were unlikely to be met unless efforts to reduce the gap between rich and poor were dramatically and rapidly scaled up. He stressed the fact that, whilst there had been improvements in some indicators, the disease burden for both communicable and non-communicable diseases still remained high, and that the poor carried a disproportionate burden of disease (United Nations, 2002). 'Long-term and upstream' as opposed to 'short-term and downstream' are principles guiding all SDE's activities.

CASE STUDY – SOUTH AFRICAN ECONOMIC GROWTH

The recent electricity shortage in South Africa is a typical example of unsustainable development. For many decades the South African economy was distributed amongst 9.1 per cent of the population. This was reflected in the decade prior to 1994, when economic growth averaged less than 1 per cent a year. Following the April 1994 transition to democratic government, the economy opened up and there was full engagement by the whole population. This resulted in an annual economic growth of over 4 per cent since September 1999 – the longest period of economic expansion in the country's recorded history.

Apparently, in 1997 the South African government was informed by the electricity provider that at this rate of economic growth, the electricity generation system would soon be vulnerable. The sustained growth, coupled with the rapid industrialisation and mass electrification programme of the last decade, finally led in January 2008 to demand for electricity outstripping supply. This is threatening to undermine efforts towards further economic growth, as signified by temporary power cuts in some gold mines around the Gauteng province.

CONCLUSION

Clearly, economic growth has the potential to address determinants of health such as poverty and employment and to promote general improvement in the standards of living. However, unless there are efforts to minimise environmental degradation, uneven distribution of resources and uneven access to the opportunities for development technologies, the growth is unlikely to last.

FURTHER READING

United Nations (1992) 'Agenda 21', in *Report of the United Nations*. Rio de Janeiro: United Nations.

United Nations (1997) *Programme for the Further Implementation of Agenda 21*. New York: United Nations.

World Health Organization (2005) *Sustainable Development and Healthy Environments: Highlights 2004: Protecting Human Health through Scientific Evidence, Reasonable Caution and Strategic Partnerships*. Geneva: WHO.

15 Health Literacy: The Public Health Perspective

Mike Horah and Mzwandile (Andi) Mabhala

key concepts
in public health

DEFINITION

Originally, literacy was considered to be the capacity to read, write and have basic numeric skills (Kickbusch, 2001; Pleasant and Kuruvilla, 2008). It has now been established that literacy is much more than that: it involves culture, individual empowerment and community development. The current literature recognises that there are two forms of literacy: general literacy and health literacy. The definition proposed by the WHO (World Health Organization, 1998) and popularised by Nutbeam (1998) reflected this broad view of literacy:

> Health literacy represents the cognitive and social skills which determine the motivation and ability of individuals to gain access to, understand and use information in ways which promote and maintain good health. (Nutbeam, 2000: 265)

KEY POINTS

- Health literacy is much more than the ability to read and write.
- The debate about general literacy as a key determinant of health tends to centre on income and income distribution, employment, working conditions and the social environment.
- While both health literacy and general literacy have important effects on social, economic and health development, there are subtle differences.
- High literacy levels do not guarantee that people will respond to health promotion and communication activities.

DISCUSSION

Health literacy has long been associated with educational attainment. The assumption has been that higher educational attainment translates to high health literacy, and thus the better chances of good health and greater wellbeing. This linkage between educational attainment and health was first reported in Black's report in 1980; it has since been documented in several reports, health policy documents and research articles. As noted earlier both health literacy and general literacy have important effects on social, economic and health development, however there are subtle differences between the two strands. The debate about general literacy as a key determinant of health tends to centre on income and income distribution, employment, working conditions and the social environment. This debate is supported by evidence that indicates that high levels of illiteracy contribute significantly to the disease burden of poor communities and countries, and reinforce health and economic inequalities. However, it has now been established that while general literacy is an important determinant of health, it is not sufficient to address the major health challenges facing developing and developed societies.

The current debate about health literacy is grounded in Nutbeam's assertion 'that high literacy levels (assessed in terms of ability to read and write) are not a guarantee that a person will respond in a desired way to health promotion and communication activities' (Nutbeam, 2000: 269).

The public health perspective makes connections between health literacy, health promotion and social marketing of public health interventions, and connects health literacy with education and empowerment (Pleasant and Kuruvilla, 2008). It recognises health literacy as a barrier to the 'fully engaged scenario' described in the Wanless Report (HM Treasury, 2002), as people with low levels of health literacy may have insufficient access to information to make sound judgements about health and its determinants. This view maintains that health literacy enables people to make sound health decisions in the context of everyday life:

- at home;
- in the community;
- at the workplace;
- in the healthcare system;
- in the marketplace;
- in the political arena.

A critical empowerment strategy is to increase people's control over their health, their ability to seek out information and their ability to take responsibility. The public health perspective is based on the assumption that individuals vary in the degree to which they exercise their health literacy skills – as service users and patients, as consumers of food and other products and services, as family members, as householders, as employees and as citizens. They also have different needs at different stages of their lives.

It is easy, but not necessarily accurate, to assume that people of significant educational attainment will also have high health literacy levels: Yet even those with high educational attainment can be faced with considerable demands on their health literacy, for example on being diagnosed with a serious or complex medical condition. Patients and families often receive volumes of information about their condition and treatment options, and are expected to interpret and understand basic health information and services, to have the competence to use such information and services to make decisions regarding informed consent, and to negotiate their treatment outcomes.

Similarly, the public health perspective considers diffusion and use of knowledge as a prerequisite for changes in attitudes and behaviours that lead to better health (Kickbusch, 2001). However, finding a diagnostic test for a person's health literacy that is suitable for the public health perspective is often a problem, though there are some tests for measuring patient literacy in a clinical setting. The Rapid Estimate of Adult Literacy in Medicine (REALM) measures the ability to read from a list of words of increasing difficulty (Gordon, 2002). The Test of Functional Health Literacy in Adults (TOFHLA) tests a patient's ability to read passages and phrases in a healthcare setting. These are in sharp contrast to the range of skills a public health approach defines as health literacy (Kickbusch, 2001). This approach sees acquisition of health knowledge as an integral part of health literacy, rather than a separate outcome (Pleasant and Kuruvilla, 2008).

A study in Glasgow used REALM to test the health literacy of patients with rheumatoid arthritis. Of 123 patients, 21 were assessed as having functional illiteracy. There were no differences in the ages, disease durations or drugs prescribed between the two groups. Functionally illiterate patients had three times as many outpatient visits and visited twice as many hospital departments. However, these tests look at only one skill set – reading – and in a clinical setting. Numeracy, ITC skills and the ability to access, comprehend and act on a wider range of non-clinical health information is just as important.

Educational outcome is a good proxy for health literacy – and more specifically for poor or low health literacy – and the education sector is a rich source of data:

- In the UK approximately 16 per cent of adults in England have literacy skills lower than that attained by the average 11-year-old.
- 46 per cent of adults have similarly low numeracy skills.
- Over 15 million adults have difficulty in calculating times in the 24 hour clock, and in reading scales.
- More than 5 million find it difficult to follow simple instructions, complete basic health forms, and explain straightforward feelings and symptoms over the phone.

A 1970 birth year cohort study looked at this group at age 33. Comparison of those who were disengaged at school and had no GCSE qualifications with those who did (Davis, 1993) revealed:

- smoking rates 4.7 times higher in women and 3.5 times higher in men;
- rates of heavy drinking 1.5 times higher;
- rates of taking exercise less than once a week 1.5 times higher;
- depression rates 2.4 times higher for women and two times higher for men;
- back pain rates 1.3 times higher in men;
- migraine rates 1.3 times higher in women;

In England the Department of Education and Skills has launched Skills for Life, the national strategy for improving the literacy, language and numeracy (LLN) skills of adults, providing millions of learning opportunities. While focused on improving skills for employment and on redressing the accumulated legacy of poor educational outcomes and the continued entry into adulthood of young people whose LLN skills are poor, it indirectly addresses poor health literacy among adults.

CASE STUDY

Maureen, a 23-year-old woman, has recently discovered that she is pregnant with her first baby. Maureen is unemployed, a heavy smoker and overweight. Irene, a community midwife, has been assigned to pay regular visits to minimise complications to Maureen's pregnancy. The community midwifery team decided to deliver a comprehensive public health package aimed at addressing all the identified health needs. Irene gave frequent brief advice on each subject mentioned above, followed by simple written material.

One day Irene came to visit Maureen and found that Maureen had missed a very important appointment with a consultant and did not inform the practice that she wasn't going to make it. Irene expressed disappointment with Maureen's lack of compliance with the advice, only to find that Maureen was honestly unaware of any appointment. She was extremely embarrassed to indicate to the community midwife that she could not read or write, and therefore had not really understood any of the written instructions given to her.

CONCLUSION

This chapter has taken a very brief overview of health literacy from the perspective of the wider determinants of health and wellbeing, and has deliberately focused on public health aspects. The emphasis has been that the importance of improving the health literacy of citizens even in mature first world societies like the UK should never be under-estimated. It is a key element of reducing inequalities in health and in empowering people to take charge of their own health.

FURTHER READING

Nutbeam, D. (2000) 'Health literacy as a public health goal: a challenge for contemporary health education and communication strategies into the 21st century', *Health Promotion International*, 15(3): 259–67.

Osbourne, H. (2005) *Health Literacy from A–Z. Practical Ways to Communicate your Health Message*. London: Jones and Bartlett.

16 Public Health and the Media

Pat Clarke

DEFINITION

Mass media have been described as 'any printed or audio-visual material designed to reach a mass audience. This includes newspapers, magazines, radio, television, billboards, exhibition displays, posters and leaflets' (Naidoo and Wills, 2000: 242). Indeed there may be many interpretations of what the mass media are, depending on individual contexts. The media have evolved to become more international than national, and include examples such as the internet; public health messages using the internet can be seen by anyone with access anywhere in the world. This expansion provides opportunities for public health as well as challenges; however, the objectives of mass media and public health rarely converge (Payne and Schulte, 2003).

Most public health initiatives are influenced by elements of mass media, and the effects of mass media may have a positive or negative impact on behaviour change. The following definition encapsulates the concept:

> Mass media resources can be seen as a means of improving current persuasive health-promotional encounters and influencing hitherto unaffected and unreachable audiences. (Whitehead, 2000: 814)

KEY POINTS

- Opportunities and challenges of the media.
- Ethics and the media.
- Conflict between the public health and mass media agendas.

DISCUSSION

Opportunities and challenges of the media

The mass media can reach a large number of people very quickly, can also contact the 'hard to reach' and are relatively cheap based on cost per person, compared to face-to-face methods; an example of this is the internet. However, unlike face-to-face methods which enable two-way communication, messages cannot be tailored to meet individual needs. Mass media can also remind the public about the effects of health-damaging behaviour, for example via programmes on alcohol consumption, or smoking bans. In contrast, soap operas such as *Coronation Street* project alcohol consumption as an enjoyable pastime. Soap operas can prompt behaviour change (Naidoo and Wills, 2000), but this may not reflect the public health agenda; indeed some people may perceive the actors as role models.

Five models have been identified concerning how the mass media affect behaviour change: hypodermic syringe, aerosol effect, two-step model, use and gratification model, and the cultural effects model (Naidoo and Wills, 2000). More than one approach may be used simultaneously in any one campaign. Further change may be due to other drivers, e.g. personal tragedy or sudden change in health status.

The 'hypodermic syringe' model (Tones and Green, 2004) is where a message is cascaded out to a large population; if the desired effect is not achieved, the message is intensified until it is. An example is the 'Back to Sleep' media campaign following the death of Anne Diamond's baby in 1991 (Fleming et al., 1996), which resulted in an immediate change in behaviour and subsequently reduced the incidence of cot death.

In the 'aerosol effect', while some information may produce the desired effect, much has little or no effect (Mendelsohn, 1968, cited in Naidoo and Wills, 2000). An example is the media campaign on obesity, where some of the information is effective but much of the target audience is not reached.

The 'two step model' (Katz and Lazarsfeld, 1955, cited in Naidoo and Wills, 2000) insists that mass media initiatives need to be followed by methods which tailor information to individual needs: examples include smoking cessation, tailoring the information to individual needs and supporting people through the behaviour change. Mass media in isolation from other methods will not result in behaviour change.

The 'use and gratification model' (Naidoo and Wills, 2000) suggests that the audience interprets the part of the health message that best aligns with their individual need, thus selecting what is most important to them. It directly conflicts with the hypodermic syringe model. While media messages about chocolates or flowers can be captivating, health messages arouse feelings of 'being controlled' or 'the nanny state', restricting enjoyment from making the prescribed change.

Finally the cultural effects model (Naidoo and Wills, 2000) suggests that the media creates an environment where values and beliefs are determined by the content of the media messages relating to health and illness. Conversely, it could be argued that pre-existing values and beliefs are challenged by the media messages. Examples of this could be the changing attitudes towards smoking, or towards drinking and driving. However, it could be argued that a number of drivers including the mass media have caused this change.

Ethics and the media

Trying to create a healthier society using the mass media can in itself create ethical dilemmas (Katz et al., 2000). Whilst many ethical dilemmas have no right or wrong answer, one must consider what resources will be committed to any particular public health initiative. In terms of ethics this decision may mean that priority is given to one area of public health over another; it is vital that these decisions can be justified in terms of benefits for the majority (Caulfield, 2006).

Arguably, the smoking ban from July 2007 impinges on individual autonomy. Mass media – television, posters and leaflets – were widely used to promote this ban. Conversely, it could be said that 'one man's freedom is another man's prison', i.e. the known effects of passive smoking may reduce opportunities to socialise.

A further example of the ethical implications of the mass media is the AIDS programme scheduled to be broadcast by the BBC in the 1980s and banned by the government at the time for fear of reprisals (Goodman, 2002). It could be argued that this decision was based on the ethical principle of non-maleficence. Based on what we know about AIDS, it may be ethically difficult to defend that decision today.

Conflict between the public health and mass media agendas

Those using the mass media to convey health messages must consider that the overall aim of journalism can be the readers' 'right to know' as opposed to 'need to know' (Berg, 2005a). Indeed, competition for news items means that public health items may take second place (Berg, 2005b), possibly because they are difficult to sensationalise.

Challenges for those using mass media as a single vehicle for public health include the following:

- It is more difficult to target a specific audience.
- They are not person-centred.
- It is difficult to know how the message has been interpreted, if at all.
- There is no opportunity for the target audience to clarify any part of the message received.
- They are mostly limited to those who speak English and have no visual impairment or auditory problems.
- It is difficult to measure effect of the message.

These, coupled with lack of understanding of the characteristics of the target group, can make it difficult to evaluate the effectiveness of public health information when using mass media to disseminate the messages.

Soap operas have played a role in providing information about public health issues: for example the 'smoking ban' was included as part of a *Coronation Street* storyline. However, the danger of using this approach can be the creation of stereotypes. On the other hand, the main part of the set is a 'public house' and many of the storylines portray alcohol consumption as an enjoyable regular habit, albeit not one in line with current public health messages.

CASE STUDY

Two case studies will be looked at, demonstrating the contrasting effects of the media on public health.

Scenario 1

In 1990 the public raised concerns about the possibility of bovine spongiform encephalitis (BSE) being transferred to humans through the consumption of beef. The government decided to help reduce anxiety in the general population by putting forward a minister (John Gummer) to give his child a beefburger; the reassured population would then supposedly continue to eat beef. Research later demonstrated that the disease agent could be transferred to humans in the form of Creutzfeldt-Jakob Disease (CJD). This resulted in the public losing confidence in the government and feeling that the public health agenda was not based on their interests.

- Consider the ethical implications of this approach to public health.
- Consider the evidence base supporting this public health message.
- Consider the implications of this type of initiative for future public health messages.

Scenario 2

On the other hand, the annual drink driving media campaign over the Christmas period brings the dangers of drink driving to the attention of the public. The aim is to reduce morbidity and mortality on the roads and reduce alcohol consumption to safer levels. A series of advertisements appears on the television and in the newspapers, and it is hoped that the ongoing reminders of the dangers will result in a decline in the number of people driving under the influence of alcohol.

- Consider the type of advertising used in this campaign.
- Has this campaign been effective and if so why?
- Are there any implications to this type of advertising?

CONCLUSION

Using mass media as the vehicle for promoting public health assumes the public has a high level understanding of the current health issues. It is necessary to consider the relationship between social marketing, health literacy and ethical issues when considering the use of mass media for public health messages.

While the mass media provide the opportunity to disseminate health messages, it must be remembered that the media are based on attracting large audiences and large profits, but not all public health messages attract large audiences or make profits. In order to achieve this, mass media often sensationalise stories (Berg, 2005a). Consequently there is a great danger that the messages will be adapted to ensure the mass media agenda is met, resulting in the main points of the public health message being lost. Those hoping to use mass media for public health messages need to be clear on the strengths and challenges of this method.

FURTHER READING

Seale, C. (2003) *Media and Health*. London: Sage.
World Health Organization (2005) *Effective Media Communication during Public Health Emergencies – a WHO Handbook*. Geneva: WHO.

17 Local Strategies for Public Health Implementation

Graham Holroyd

DEFINITION

There has been an increasing emphasis on 'engaging with communities', 'collaboration', 'partnership' and 'joint working' of late. This is particularly prevalent in the arena of public health (Earle, 2007), and has increased significantly with the formation and implementation of the policies of the New Labour government. The reason for this, it is suggested, is to enhance the effectiveness of the impact of the policies. One of the aims of these policies is to reduce social and fiscal inequalities, and ultimately to alleviate the effects of poverty on health by fostering social inclusion and engendering a sense of community (Centre for Urban and Community Research, 2005). The suggested 'tools' or 'ways of working' are evident in the concepts of 'social capital' and 'capacity building', which could potentially also be considered as a cure-all panacea for societal ills, by public health policy-makers at both national and local levels (Gibson, 2007).

KEY POINTS

- There is an emerging agenda of community engagement in public health.
- The concept of the changing nature of the community needs to be considered.
- Effective ways of engaging with communities should be developed.
- Some communities may be difficult to work with.
- People are leading atomised lives, so engagement is a challenge.
- There is a need for an effective evaluation tool.
- Participation at local level is crucial to meeting local public health need.

It is worth considering that the word 'community' is becoming more widely used and therefore increasingly difficult to define. Williams (1988) suggests that its usage has developed, and been (mis) appropriated over a number of years. It is overlaid with a plethora of meanings. Williams also suggests that it is one word that never appears to be used unfavourably, and can evoke, not always appropriately, feelings of closeness, warmth and belonging. Hawtin et al. (1999) concur with this, suggesting that:

> In reality, communities are not always comfortable homogenous entities. They are crosscut by a variety of divisions – race, gender, and class – and contain a multitude of groups whose interests may conflict with each other. In the most divided communities, these conflicts may be played out violently or through such behaviour as racial harassment. (Hawtin et al., 1999: 34)

The word community also suggests a common bond between individuals, groups or sections of the population, and subsequently a commonality of understanding of the public health needs of that community. Professionally defined geographical areas or localities may also define a community, varying in size from a single street to a neighbourhood, for example an administratively defined area, as in the case of Primary Care Trusts. There are, however, other characteristics which may define a community: the individuals who live there, for example, may define a community more appropriately. These characteristics may include a sense of inclusiveness, and belonging to that community. Conversely, it may also mean, to some, exclusion by members of that same community. The characteristics of community may be based upon, for example, ethnicity, gender, religion, or a mutually shared issue or problem. The concept and reality of community between professional and lay people, or policy-makers and recipients, are also vastly different, and will have implications for locally delivered public health. Do these issues help us in some way to understand the complexities of engaging with members of communities and developing and implementing public health policies?

Are we clear as to how and why we should engage with communities effectively, and how we encourage members of communities to participate fully in decision-making regarding public health issues? Community participation doesn't just happen, it is initiated and works best when a number of different interests willingly come together, formally or informally, to achieve some common purpose (Wilcox, 1994). Community engagement for partnership work, and ultimately policy formation and implementation, is not about manipulating or educating people, nor is it about placating a group of handpicked tokenistic 'worthies' and placing them on committees or in focus groups (Holroyd, 2002). How do we engage effectively with communities?

There is a need to explore the notions of collaborative working, and in this respect that 'social capital' and 'capacity building', the bywords of community engagement, are not uni-dimensional: they are in fact activities that address a continuum, from micro to macro level, (Jackson et al., 1997). The myth and reality of community participation in the implementing of local public health policies also need to be considered and the contested, ever-changing characteristics of communities discussed. The importance of harnessing, or at least recognising the synergy between the community, state and social institutions as a way of reducing social inequalities and increasing social inclusion will also need to be considered. In conclusion, the difficulty of evaluating endeavours in this area will be reflected upon.

Partnerships for public health policy implementation

The potential for alliances and partnership work with all stakeholders is fundamental to the success of recent government public health policies, and will be even more so in the future (National Audit Office, 2004). The Local Government and Public Involvement in Health Bill, introduced to parliament in December 2006 (DH, 2006), reinforces this. It contained a number of measures relating to the role of local government as well as the involvement of local communities. One of the measures the bill introduced was the establishment of Local Involvement Networks (LINks), which replace patients' forums, and the Commission for Patient and Public Involvement in Health in 2008. The bill also clarifies and strengthens the existing duty on NHS bodies to involve and consult with patients and the public in the planning and provision of services, in effect, to work in a 'Healthy Alliance'.

The term 'Healthy Alliances' came to prominence following the publication of the Health of the Nation strategy (DH, 1992). *Our Healthier Nation* (DH, 1998a) also advocated that a wide range of agencies should be involved in the implementation of policies to deliver local healthcare, and that a multi-agency approach would be of benefit to all. *Our Healthier Nation* also stated that through Primary Care Groups (later to be Primary Care Trusts) local people should be involved in decision-making too. This approach has been reiterated in the White Paper, *Choosing Health* (DH, 2004b). Here, the emphasis is placed on agencies involved in public health, and health and social care, to 're-engage with their constituents', i.e. members of communities. In the context of working effectively with communities, and encouraging participation we could consider the core principles of a Community Development approach.

The Community Development approach suggests that community participation is an ongoing and organic process. Community Development can be summarised simply as an approach towards creating structures and fora to facilitate the sharing of information. Hawtin et al., (1999) suggest that its ultimate aim is to respond to the needs of the particular community, thus facilitating more 'ownership' by the community. Through these means, it is suggested that individuals, groups or organisations can become engaged in the consultation process and ultimately help formulate policies.

In some instances, for example public health policy development, members of communities may have the opportunity to become actively involved in a project or programme, and have an effect on the outcome of the decisions made. The underlying principle of alliances, partnerships and working collaboratively with the community is based on the principles of empowerment and the redistribution of power (Wilcox, 1994). This is undertaken through negotiation between community members and those who have decision-making powers. But how easy is it to work collaboratively?

Collaborative working

Inclusive and collaborative ways of working have become more prevalent in all areas of public services; however, this is increasingly evident in the arena of public health (Statham, 2000). The government has encouraged many different forms of collaborative ways of working. Examples include the Home Office Community Cohesion Strategy, the Neighbourhood Renewal Unit, and most recently in health, as detailed in *Choosing Health* (DH, 2004b). A number of other non-governmental agencies are also contributing to the debate; these include, most recently, the British Urban Regeneration Programme (BURA) and the Economic and Social Research Council (ESRC).

CASE STUDY

The ESRC has recently undertaken research with the University of Essex into the effects of participation on local democracy and decision-making. This research has also considered the relationship between participation by members of communities and the effect this has on health (ESRC, 2004). The reasons for working in a collaborative way with communities are manifold, but have two common elements: reinforcing the common interests of the community, and making services more relevant to locally defined need. This collaborative and inclusive way of working, it is suggested, also helps in reducing social and health inequalities (Whitehead, 1995).

In some way, though, it could be argued that this initiative – the notion of engaging with communities, and increasingly the word 'community' itself – may be used as a spray-on solution to solve complex social problems (Minkler, 1997).

CONCLUSION

There is a need to reflect on the merit of local involvement or community engagement in policy-making and implementation. As yet, (El Ansari et al., 2001b) suggests that there is little or no evidence of the effectiveness, or an effective tool for measuring the worth, of engaging with communities. As this way of working becomes more prevalent in the area of public health, there is an urgent need for this to be addressed.

This chapter has highlighted some of the challenges and opportunities for all involved in the implementation of public health strategies at local level to reflect on the most appropriate way of working, and to harness the potential synergy between citizens, individually and collectively, and agents of the state, for the benefit of all.

FURTHER READING

Economic and Social Research Council (2004) *Participation and Democracy – A Health Check for British Democracy*. Swindon: ESRC Publications.
National Audit Office (2004) *Getting Citizens Involved: Community Participation in Neighbourhood Renewal*. London: National Audit Office.

18 Ethics of Public Health

Jill McCarthy

DEFINITION

Ethics is generally regarded as the study of the *values* and *customs* of a person or group or people (Crisp, 1998). Ethics is concerned with morality; deciding upon the right action and making the right choices in situations which arise. Public health ethics can be defined as the standards and values which guide actions designed to promote the health and wellbeing of a population and prevent injury and ill health (Gostin, 2002). Ethics in public health differs from ethics in healthcare in that with the former there is concern about making the right choices and actions for a shared group or community as opposed to an individual

(Coughlin, 2006). It is a relatively new area of ethics and, as such, the body of knowledge is still growing and being developed (Bradley and Burls, 2002; Goldenburg, 2005). A code of ethics for public health has not yet been formulated, primarily because the wide range of practitioners and practices involved in work for public health has resulted in the field being highly eclectic and at times conflicting (Beaglehole and Bonita, 1997).

KEY POINTS

- Ethics in public health is concerned with community wellbeing.
- Ethics in public health differs from ethics in healthcare.
- Public health ethics is a relatively new area.
- There is no code of ethics specific to public health workers.

DISCUSSION

Public health ethics can be viewed from two distinct perspectives: the ethics of public health workers or *professional ethics*; and ethics within public health theory and practice or *applied ethics* (Gostin, 2000). Both of these perspectives are equally important and although they are patently intertwined they can be unpicked for the purpose of scrutiny in order to enrich knowledge and understanding of the issues involved.

Professional ethics

Professional ethics within public health is concerned with the moral behaviour and actions of the various professionals employed in this field (Rogers, 2004). Professionals working within public health have a duty to act in the best interests of their client groups and should behave in a virtuous manner at all times. However, without an ethical code of conduct to refer to this can occasionally prove problematic. Consider the case of a nurse whose role includes public health work, who is advising a client undergoing radiotherapy for breast cancer. The client cannot tolerate a seat belt across her chest due to the sensitivity of her skin in this area. When advising the client, does the nurse consider the benefits to the community she works with in regard to seat belt legislation or the rights of the individual who is in pain and discomfort?

At times public health work appears to oppose the autonomy and welfare of individuals, and the professional must consider if their duty of care is to the community they serve or to the individuals they are involved in working with. The word community is in itself vague and unclear; there may be various groups within a community all of whom can present with differing and conflicting interests. Action groups keen to change current public health practices may have clear and well thought out rationales for their opinions, and practitioners need to be knowledgeable and informed in order to put the public health viewpoint across effectively. It is the ethical duty of a public health professional to aim to bring about the greatest good, in terms of health benefits and disease prevention, for the greatest number of people and they should be guided by this principle (Buchanan, 2000). This is not to say that the importance of individual autonomy and freedom should be sacrificed, but that the importance of citizenship, community and partnerships should be recognised and protected, wherever possible (Gostin, 2002).

Applied ethics

Applied ethics is concerned with the ethical theory and practice of public health work and less with the moral behaviour of the professionals concerned. It is interested in ethical reasoning in order to produce public health policies and practices of optimum benefit to the communities these professionals serve. This covers a diverse range of areas including demography, disease prevention, epidemiology, healthcare, health education, health promotion, sanitation and social care. The ethical issues involved centre upon such topics as unwittingly discriminating against groups of people while attempting to benefit the health or welfare of a community; finding the correct balance between autonomy and paternalism; acting in an advocacy role for a community which is powerless or oppressed; balancing decreasing budgets with increasing health needs. For example, consider the tax burden placed on tobacco which is generally regarded as a tactic to discourage smoking and, therefore, benefit the health of the nation. However, when one considers that smokers account for a disproportionably large number of people in lower social classes IV and V (HM Treasury, 2004) it can also be regarded as a tax burden predominantly aimed at the poorer people in society. Obviously, the government considers this tax is justified, but can the underlying implications be regarded as ethically sound?

CASE STUDY

James is a 48-year-old man who suffers from sensitivity to certain chemicals and foodstuffs. Often this results in severe allergic reactions and, sometimes, life-threatening anaphylactic shock. James has been patch tested for these sensitivities and has been diagnosed with a positive allergy to over 100 foodstuffs and food additives, including fluoride. In the borough where James lives, the water supply has fluoride added to it at source with the intention of minimising and preventing tooth decay and caries in the population it serves. James finds it extremely inconvenient and expensive to use bottled water for all his hygiene and dietary needs and has subsequently contacted his council to discuss this matter. It is James' intention to persuade the council that it is unethical to add chemicals to drinking water without the permission of every householder, as James considers this a flouting of individual human rights. Moreover, he believes that even if the benefits for dental health from fluoridation are founded, sources of fluoride are numerous and easily attainable without adding it to the water supply.

The council refers James to the Strategic Health Authority (SHA) for his area as it is responsible for determining either the initiation or cessation of water fluoridation under the direction of the Water (Fluoridation) Act 1985. James contacts his local SHA and discusses this matter with an official who is sympathetic to his case, although she makes it clear that they are unable to make changes to the water supply as, after wide public debate, the SHA decided that the benefits to the population as a whole far outweighed the disadvantages to a limited number of individuals such as James. She further states that the practice of fluoridation of water has been endorsed by the World Health Organization (2002), the British Medical Association, the Faculty of Public Health Medicine and the British Dental Association, due to evidence from numerous studies conducted worldwide which demonstrate that fluoridated drinking water reduces tooth decay and has no adverse effects (Medical Research Council, 2002). She states that she will forward information to James in regard to the decision to fluoridate the water in his area.

James receives the information pack from the SHA which consists of several reports including a summary of the Independent Inquiry into Inequalities in Health (DH, 1998a) which states that water fluoridation should decrease inequalities in dental caries between geographical areas and between socio-economic groups. James is interested to note that there is also opposition to his view that fluoridation is not ethical practice and he realises that there is a conflict of interests between the rights of individuals and the public health rights of a community. This situation is neatly summed up in the literature sent to James by the inclusion of a statement from Professor John Harris (1998):

The right to fluoride free water is not a basic civil right ... It is not a right which affects the ability of individuals to make autonomous choices ... In considering the ethics of fluoridation ... we should ask not are we entitled to impose fluoridation on unwilling people, but are the unwilling people entitled to impose the risks, damage and costs of failure to fluoridate on the community at large.

CONCLUSION

Public health ethics is concerned with bringing about the greatest benefits in terms of health and wellbeing to a population, while attempting to minimise any disruption to the rights and autonomy of the individuals concerned. It is also concerned with guiding the decisions and moral behaviours of the various professionals who are involved in public health work. It is not a clear-cut area and there are no correct answers to the ethical dilemmas which present themselves in this field of work. Professionals in public health work often face complex problems which include diminishing budgets, conflicting interests, and tensions by interest groups keen to influence public health programmes. In order to meet these challenges successfully, continuing education programmes and ongoing development of public health ethics are needed in order to inform and structure this burgeoning area of work.

FURTHER READING

Bradley, P. and Burls, A. (2002) *Ethics in Public and Community Health*. London: Routledge.

Gostin, L.O. (2002) *Public Health Law and Ethics: A Reader*. New York: University of California Press.

ethics of public health

19 Social Exclusion and Stigma

Elizabeth Mason-Whitehead

DEFINITION

The origins of the word stigma are to be found in the Greek language (the plural is stigmata). Stigma traditionally referred to the cuts or burns imprinted on the skin of slaves, traitors and criminals. Stigma, although a term which is rooted in classical civilisation, is also one that has expanded and adapted to the changing norms and constructs of centuries of cultural and social upheavals. The most celebrated definition of stigma used is that put forward by the Canadian Erving Goffman:

> While the stranger is present before us, evidence can arise of his possessing an attribute which makes him different from others in the category of persons available for him to be, and of a less desirable kind – in the extreme a person who is quite thoroughly bad, or dangerous, or weak. He is thus reduced in our minds from a whole and usual person to a tainted and discounted one. Such an attribute is a stigma ... (Goffman, 1961: 12)

Curtis's interpretation of stigma moves the definition forward to address the complex societies of the twenty-first century: 'Stigma is expressed by a majority emphasizing non-productivity, dangerousness and personal culpability of excluded groups (Curtis, 2004: 77).

Social exclusion is a term frequently used in political discussions on poverty and social upheaval and may be the result of being stigmatised. For a contemporary definition of social exclusion readers are directed to the interpretation put forward by the London School of Economics' Centre for Analysis of Social Exclusion (CASE):

> An individual is socially excluded if a) he or she is geographically resident in society, b) he or she cannot participate in activities in that society and c) he or she would like to so participate, but is prevented from doing so by factors beyond his or her control. (Richardson and le Grande, 2002)

KEY POINTS

- Stigma and social exclusion are intrinsic realities of society.
- An 'attribute' that carries a stigma in one society may not do so elsewhere. For example female circumcision is an illegal practice in the UK.
- Most people have been victims and perpetrators of stigma; for example bullying at work or racial prejudice.
- There are conditions and attributes carrying a deep-rooted stigma that does not always shift with changing times, e.g. leprosy.
- Stigma is a fluid experience. Young unmarried women who became pregnant a century ago were undoubtedly shunned, hidden away and often forced to have illegal abortions or give their babies up for adoption. Society, with its changing norms, has largely accepted teenage pregnant women as members of society (Whitehead, 2000).
- Every generation has a new wave of stigmata to manage. From the beginning of this century examples include obesity, sex workers, migrant workers and children born to HIV-positive parents.
- Perpetrators of stigma can cause profound significant emotional pain, which may last for life.
- Stigmatising an individual or group of people can lead to social exclusion, for example of sex workers.
- Public health workers are ideally placed to develop policies which seek to address and overcome stigma and social exclusion.

Erving Goffman remains the leading and most influential theorist on stigma; others include Edward Jones and Graham Scambler.

DISCUSSION

This discussion is intended to provide the reader with an overview of stigma and social exclusion which entwines the academic perspective with practical applications. The following sections should prompt debate and further reading.

Stigma and social exclusion in context

The decision for a person to accept or reject another because of a perceived difference is dependent upon a range of human experiences, such as cultural norms, the influences laid down in childhood; peer pressure, education, relationships and self-esteem. For example,

social exclusion and stigma

paedo-philes are stigmatised and socially excluded because society considers their behaviour abhorrent, breaking all 'rules' of trust, common decency and inflicting pain upon one of the most vulnerable groups in society, children. In every sense, paedophilia is an extreme state and generally speaking public health workers will be confronted by issues that have the potential to carry stigma depending upon the condition, the time and the place. At the time of writing this chapter, the UK is faced with another outbreak of foot and mouth disease and the public health consequences for some people will be significant – not so much the fear of a physical illness in the human population, but the effect this potential epidemic will have on the mental health of farmers and their families: suicide in the farming community was a serious and disturbing outcome of foot and mouth in 2001. For the families that are left, the burden that their parent, child, spouse or partner has committed suicide because of the stress may leave them feeling stigmatised and socially excluded. Society may view suicide as route out and a failing in responsibility. The *transfer of stigma* to the next of kin demonstrates the power of stigma over the significant people associated with the victim.

Categorising stigma

When we consider who in society is stigmatised an eclectic group of people come to mind, such as those living in poverty, criminals, those who look different and those who behave oddly – the list seems endless. Erving Goffman, best known for his work on stigma, in his seminal text *Stigma* (1963) describes three groups of stigma which categorise all those who are perceived as carrying a 'discrediting attribute'. The use of words reflects the time when they were written and you are asked to be aware of this when reading them:

- Abominations of the body – various physical deformities.
- Blemishes of individual character perceived as weak will, domineering or unnatural passions, treacherous and rigid beliefs and dishonesty.
- Tribal stigma of race, nation, and religion, these being stigma that can be transmitted through lineages and equally contaminate all members of the family.

Although our language has changed, these broad categorisations continue to be used.

Understanding stigma from a perspective of affective psychology

In the 1980s Edward Jones gave stigma a fresh perspective and building upon the work of Goffman (and others) moved stigma from sociology to social psychology. In doing so he and his co-writers identified a conceptual framework of stigma, which they described as a mental strategy to deal with the implications of stigma. Their six dimensions of stigma are:

- Concealability – can an individual hide his or her stigma?
- Course – What are the social outcomes of the social stigma?
- Disruptiveness – how does the stigma hamper social interaction?
- Aesthetic qualities – are the signs of stigma upsetting?
- Origin – Who if anyone is to blame for the stigma?
- Peril – How serious is the stigma?

These dimensions of stigma are useful pointers in assessing whether an individual feels stigmatised (Whitehead, 2000).

Working towards social inclusion

In 1997 the then Labour government set up the Social Exclusion Unit, which is concerned with addressing society's most difficult problems, for example poverty, crime, unemployment and health inequalities. A report from the Social Exclusion Task Force (2006) delivered an 'Action Plan on Social Exclusion' putting forward headings for change:

- Better identification and earlier intervention.
- Systematically identifies 'what works'.
- Promoting multi-agency working.
- Personalised rights and responsibilities.
- Supportive achievement and managing under performance.

A creative initiative has been published by the Institute for Volunteering Research which advocates volunteering as way of overcoming social exclusion. In their report; *Volunteering for All: Exploring the Link between Volunteering and Social Exclusion* (2004), the institute identifies five positive outcomes when people who are socially excluded engage with volunteering. It

- is empowering;
- reduces isolation;

- increases self-worth;
- develops new skills;
- may create employment.

The model for change put forward by Mason and co-authors is a four-stage process (Figure 19.1).

Stage 1:	*Personal Beliefs:*	The catalyst for change
Stage 2:	*Primary Social Interaction:*	Example: A meeting followed by intervention
	Primary Social Intervention:	Example: New culture of awareness is developed
Stage 3:	*Secondary Social Interaction:*	Example: Education
	Secondary Social Intervention:	Example: Developing curriculum
Stage 4:	*Tertiary Social Action:*	Example: Producing work that has permanence
	Tertiary Social Intervention:	Example: Research, education, publishing, policy-making

Figure 19.1 *Stigma and social exclusion in healthcare practice: a model for change (adapted from Mason et al., 2000)*

CASE STUDY

Anna began work in an agricultural area in a part of England not used to incomers, and when she and her brother arrived in a small village to pick strawberries they were treated with some suspicion and even resentment. The brother and sister had arrived from Czechoslovakia to find work and send money home. Anna and her brother lived in a rented caravan and they often looked dishevelled and out of place. The situation was exacerbated when Anna fell on some agricultural machinery and seriously injured her leg. She was taken to the local Accident and Emergency Department and seen immediately by the nursing and medical staff. Some of the waiting patients heard Anna's foreign voice and on realising that she was a Czech agricultural worker shouted abuse at her such as, 'You're taking our jobs!' and 'Go home, gypsy!' Despite

key concepts in public health

Anna only taking jobs that local people did not want and learning English, she found that being stigmatised and socially excluded was too hurtful and both she and her brother moved away.

CONCLUSION

Stigma and social exclusion exist throughout the world's societies and most of us have been at one time or another both its perpetrators and its victims. The outcome of being stigmatised can be deeply wounding, and we may carry lifelong emotional and social scars. It is important that those working in public health have an understanding of stigma and social exclusion and the impact it has on groups of people and individuals. Intrinsic to public health should be an awareness of how certain conditions carry stigma and the challenges that this brings to all those working towards making communities healthier and safer places to live.

FURTHER READING

Curtis, S. (2004) *Health and Inequality*. London: Sage.

Mason, T., Carlisle, C., Watkins, C. and Whitehead, E. (eds) (2000) *Stigma and Social Exclusion in Healthcare*. London: Routledge.

Scambler, G. (2005) *Medical Sociology: Major Themes in Health and Social Welfare*. London: Routledge.

20 Vulnerability

Jan Hardy and Tina Barrows

DEFINITION

The term vulnerable can mean different things to different people. Originally it was derived from the Latin verb *vulnerare* which means to wound (Aday, 1993). A review of health literature reveals how often the term 'vulnerability' appears in text, yet there is no comprehensive consensus on the precise definition, which leaves it open to individual interpretation and consequently makes application to practice problematic (Costello and Haggart, 2003).

KEY POINTS

- Vulnerability is dependent upon an individual's internal and external factors.
- Vulnerability can be demonstrated within a lifecycle continuum.
- Vulnerability is closely linked with the concept of risk and susceptibility.

DISCUSSION

Vulnerability is not an unusual phenomenon; there are times in our lives when we all feel vulnerable, whether through illness or injury (Sellman, 2005) or in situations that allow us little or no control. The feeling of vulnerability is further compounded when individuals feel unsure of themselves, lack the knowledge to improve a situation or are excluded from a society that fails to identify with their circumstances.

Internal and external factors

Vulnerability has been found to be a complex changeable interaction between internal factors (self-esteem, social support networks, personal relationships and degree of health and wellbeing) and external factors (housing, finances, employment status and level of control over life circumstances) which can have a profound impact on an individual's ability to cope, compounding their feeling of vulnerability (Rose and Killien, 1983; Copp, 1986; Rogers, 1997).

The consequences of living with adverse conditions can compound one's susceptibility to developing poor health. Homeless and socially excluded individuals are at greater risk of developing both physical and mental health problems (Flaskerud and Winslow, 1998). Vulnerability can enhance feelings of inadequacy and lack of confidence in expressing any concerns regarding health matters, thereby rendering an individual or group even more vulnerable.

Lone mothers have been found to be more prone to mental health problems whereas the unemployed are found to have far-reaching problems across the health spectrum (Baker et al., 2002) including cardiovascular disease and psychological problems. Studies have been instrumental in demonstrating the consequences of vulnerability on different groups both from a physical and a psychological perspective; however, the health effects of material deprivation are rarely considered.

Vulnerability as a lifecycle continuum

Despite experiencing adverse conditions or situations, many have the capacity to cope and remain healthy. It would appear that the ability to cope is dependent on the interplay of an individual's genetic predisposition and coping mechanisms with the environment. This can dictate why some 'survive' and others fail to cope. Figure 20.1 depicts how a lifecycle continuum renders an individual vulnerable (also see Case Study).

Vulnerability within the concept of risk

Vulnerability is often used interchangeably with the concept of 'at' risk. Risk implies the presence of stressful factors in a person's environment that can be damaging to health, whilst vulnerability refers to the personal factors that interact with the environment to influence health (Rose and Killien, 1983; Rogers, 1997). Both are key factors when assessing health needs. Assessing risk in the wider context allows for a more comprehensive and overarching evaluation when determining the likelihood of an event occurring or identifying those people who may in the future go on to develop problems.

If we accept that vulnerability can mean 'susceptibility to harm' or 'risk of harm' then we must inevitably acknowledge the implications and challenges that this brings. Public health is reliant on a multidisciplinary approach in meeting health needs. This is evident at different levels, from the individual's perspective – when they are encouraged to take responsibility for their own actions and consider lifestyle choices (King's Fund, 2004a) – through to decisions taken by national and international bodies to improve the health of populations (Earle et al., 2007). Many people feel powerless to change their situation and find their circumstances are influenced by factors that are inextricably linked and often outside their control. Often an individual experiences a cascading range of problems which contribute to an already vulnerable lifestyle.

Exploring the public health issues relating to the case study will highlight how a multi-professional approach is required to address the many issues that arise.

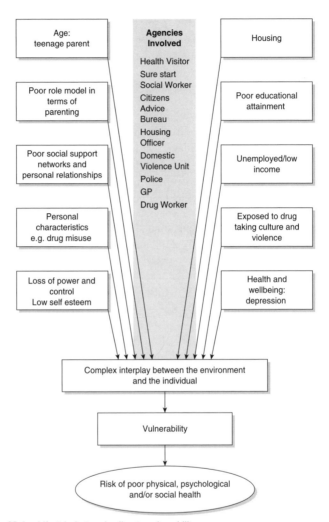

Age: teenage parent	Agencies Involved	Housing
Poor role model in terms of parenting	Health Visitor Sure start Social Worker Citizens Advice Bureau Housing Officer Domestic Violence Unit Police GP Drug Worker	Poor educational attainment
Poor social support networks and personal relationships		Unemployed/low income
Personal characteristics e.g. drug misuse		Exposed to drug taking culture and violence
Loss of power and control Low self esteem		Health and wellbeing: depression

Complex interplay between the environment and the individual

Vulnerability

Risk of poor physical, psychological and/or social health

Figure 20.1 *Lifestyle factors leading to vulnerability*

key concepts in public health

CASE STUDY

Cheryl is a 19-year-old single mother. She has two children aged 2 and 3 years. She lived with her father and stepmother until 15 years of age (her mother died when she was 7 years old). Throughout that time her experience of being parented was poor. Failing to complete her education, she ran away from home and lived rough. She took drugs spasmodically, and her personal relationships were often with violent men.

At 16 years she moved in with a boyfriend, who was violent and a drug user, and had two children with him. They were both unemployed and relied on benefits which the boyfriend used to buy drugs. They were finally evicted for non-payment of rent.

At a chance meeting with her estranged sister Cheryl was persuaded to start her life again away from her boyfriend and the violence. She stayed in her sister's overcrowded council house. She refused several housing offers due to the areas having anti-social behaviour issues and known drug issues which she felt would be a bad influence on the children.

Cheryl felt powerless to change her situation: she became withdrawn and moody. She eventually saw a GP and was diagnosed with depression.

How vulnerability compounds public health issues for some individuals

The case study highlights Cheryl's vulnerability at several stages in her life. Cheryl could be described as vulnerable from the time she lost her mother, then later when she experienced a poor role model in terms of being parented.

Becoming homeless at the age of 15 through running away from home precipitated Cheryl's journey to becoming even more vulnerable. Homelessness causes people to despair of their situation and can often lead to mental and physical illness, as demonstrated in the case study (Mason et al., 2001). The life expectancy of an individual who is homeless and sleeping rough is estimated to be 42 years, half that of the average UK citizen.

Becoming pregnant as an adolescent, according to Mulcahy (2004), magnified Cheryl's vulnerability. Teenage pregnancy has been identified as a cause and an outcome of social exclusion (Social Science Research Unit, 2005). The Social Exclusion Unit's report on *Teenage Pregnancy* (1999) identified the increased risks faced by adolescents as a consequence of teenage pregnancy such as poor health and social outcomes.

The government continues to develop policies in support of teenage parents such as Sure Start Plus, a project embraced by the Teenage Pregnancy Strategy which focused on supporting pregnant teenagers and parents. The support from the government is ongoing as regards policy: the Children Act 2004 has been instrumental in forming a cohesive legislative framework of reforms to meet the needs of children's services in order to achieve the Every Child Matters agenda which incorporates the children and young people's *National Service Framework* (DH, 2004d). Placing children's centres in areas where they are accessible for young parents and teenagers should provide those families with the support of specialised services.

Due to her poor educational achievement, Cheryl lacked the knowledge to access appropriate information on housing and accommodation which might have allowed her to make better choices concerning her own and her children's safety. Assistance can be sought under the homelessness legislation, and priority is given to families with children; however, a lengthy wait in temporary accommodation can ensue. Tackling the root cause of homelessness is an ambitious challenge. This is highlighted in the Green Paper, 'Care Matters' (DfES, 2007a), where the government acknowledges that young people in care require further support for as long as they need it in order for them to prepare themselves for living on their own and supporting themselves. The government's strategy is to encourage councils to focus on prevention of homelessness, but this can often prove difficult since people are in crisis when they seek help.

Cheryl's circumstances could be described as critical, particularly when the violence between herself and her partner increased. The government's National Action Plan on Domestic Violence (Home Office, 2005) highlights the need for increased protection and support to victims of domestic violence, and the need to be more proactive in bringing perpetrators to justice. This requires early intervention and identification of victims, changing attitudes towards the concept of domestic violence and reporting the risk of harm faced by children living with domestic violence.

Cheryl's situation was compounded by the fact that her partner was involved in drug misuse. Donaldson and Donaldson (2003) suggest that drug misusers are influenced by other factors that have led them to make the decision to use drugs, such as deprivation combined with poor educational attainment, social exclusion and lack of family support. Drug misuse can be the catalyst of deprivation and not just the end product (DH, 1998b).

Cheryl clearly identifies her feelings of powerlessness. She acknowledges that if she continues to expose her children to the violence and drug misuse already witnessed, their lives could be blighted (Newland and Cowley, 2003). Cheryl, despite feeling powerless to change her situation, does in fact demonstrate 'Power from Within' as described by Labonte and Robertson (1996), which is supported by Rissel's (1994) notion of gaining a sense of control over one's life.

Studies have found that single mothers are more likely to develop depression based on their social circumstances (Baker et al., 2002; Skärsäter, 2006). The government's strategy in relation to teenage pregnancy should go partway to identifying those individuals who are vulnerable to depression while offering the appropriate support.

CONCLUSION

Vulnerability is a complicated phenomenon. It can occur at any time in an individual's life and is a complex interplay between the environment and the individual.

FURTHER READING

Mulcahy, H. (2004) 'Vulnerable family as understood by public health nurses', *Community Practitioner*, 77: 257–60.
Scott, L. (2003) 'Vulnerability, need and significant harm: an analysis tool', *Community Practitioner*, 76: 468–73.

vulnerability

Part II
Practical Concepts

21 Assessing Public Health Need

Pat Rose

DEFINITION

In the context of public health, Health Needs Assessment (HNA) has a very specific meaning. It is defined by the National Institute for Health and Clinical Excellence (NICE, 2005: 3) as 'a systematic method for reviewing the health issues facing a population'. Thus it is the focus on the population rather than the individual that is the key attribute. NICE continues the definition by adding that its purpose is to lead to 'agreed priorities and resource allocation that will improve health and reduce inequalities'. Hawtin et al. (1999), in describing community profiling comment that needs assessment should be carried out with the active involvement of the community.

KEY POINTS

Health needs assessment:

- is focused on populations, not individuals;
- leads to agreement regarding health priorities and resource allocation;
- requires the active involvement of service users as representatives of the population.

DISCUSSION

NICE (2005) uses the work of Dahlgren and Whitehead (1991) (Figure 3.1, see p. 18) to identify the focus of health needs assessment in terms of the determinants of health of individuals, communities and society.

They acknowledge that all factors need to be addressed in order to improve both health and service delivery. However, they argue that it is only worthwhile undertaking an HNA if it will result in changes that will benefit the whole population. Clearly therefore the focus of the assessment is the general socio-economic, cultural and environmental conditions, and the social and community networks.

There have been a number of attempts to establish the nature of need. Bradshaw (1972) suggested that there are four distinct types of need (Box 21.1).

Box 21.1

Felt: individual perceptions of variations from normal health

Expressed: individuals seek help to overcome variation from normal health

Normative: the desirable standard as judged by professionals

Comparative: comparison between needs for severity, size, range of interventions, cost

---

It could be argued that, because the focus of HNA is on populations, it is the comparative need that is the business of public health professionals. For example, part of an HNA of a population may involve a comparison of mortality and morbidity as a result of heart disease in neighbouring areas. The area with the worst statistics would be judged as being in need of resources. However, the drive towards involvement of individuals in HNA means that the felt needs of service users will almost certainly be an influencing factor, with those groups expressing their needs most vocally having the greatest influence.

Endacott (1997) suggests that one attribute of the concept of need is that with it comes a responsibility to make good the deficit. Sheppard and Woodcock (1999) develop this notion to suggest that there are two approaches to understanding need. First, the familiar deficit approach: need indicates a lack of something. Secondly, however they suggest an approach which identifies need not as a deficit, but as that which resolves the deficit: the requirement to action approach. This is well illustrated by Wright (1998) who introduces the epidemiological approach to HNA. This approach assumes first that need in relation to a specific problem can be identified using estimates of incidence, prevalence and health impact (e.g. quality of life, morbidity, mortality). Secondly, it assumes that the ways in which existing services are delivered will influence the nature and extent of the need. For example, Wright describes how rates of coronary artery revascularisation and prevalence of angina were explored to assess whether use of health services reflects need. The findings were that although angina and mortality from heart disease were more common in areas with high deprivation scores, treatment by revascularisation procedures was more common in more affluent areas. This suggests that resources should be focused on ensuring that people in the deprived areas had improved access to treatment. In other words, the need that the service providers have a responsibility to meet is the requirement to improve access to treatment.

Nardi and Petr (2003) describe two conceptual frameworks which provide different points of view in relation to prioritising and directing an HNA of a population. They are the community-as-partner model and the ecological model.

Community-as-partner model is a systems-based approach in which the core system is the people who make up the community. The community is presented as consisting of nine subsystems: physical environment; community safety; transportation; health and human services; economics; education; politics; government; and recreation. Within this model it is assumed that the subsystems and core system interact in a way that affects both. Assessment of need must include an assessment of the core and all the subsystems. A partnership between all service providers and the community is the key to accurate assessment.

The underlying assumption of the ecological model is that health is influenced by the natural environment, such as location, weather and pollution, and by the built environment, including home, work, school and recreational facilities. The influences act at individual, interpersonal, organisational community and public policy levels. Determining the influence of the environment on individuals' behaviours and the influence of these behaviours on the environment is the focus of HNA.

NICE (2005: 20–47) proposes a five-step process of HNA (Box 21.2):

Box 21.2 *Five-step approach to health needs assessment (NICE, 2005)*

Step 1: Getting started

- What population?
- What are you trying to achieve?
- Who needs to be involved?
- What resources are required?
- What are the risks?

Step 2: Identifying health priorities

- Population profiling
- Gathering data
- Perceptions of needs
- Identifying and assessing health conditions and determinant factors

Step 3: Assessing a health priority for action

- Choosing health conditions and determinant factors with the most significant size and severity impact
- Determining effective and acceptable interventions and actions

Step 4: Planning for change

- Clarifying aims of intervention
- Action planning
- Monitoring and evaluation strategy
- Risk-management strategy

Step 5: Moving on/review

- Learning from the project
- Measuring impact
- Choosing the next priority

They also outline the skills that are needed in order to carry out HNA: project management; team building; partnership working; community engagement; population profiling; data collection and monitoring/ setting indicators (NICE, 2005: 50–53). A multidisciplinary team of public health professionals needs to identify who has which skills and use them accordingly to conduct an effective HNA. For example a health visitor may bring the skill of community engagement to the team, and a member of the clinical audit department would bring data collection skills.

CASE STUDY

The local population of the Primary Care Trust (PCT) is of mixed ethnicity. The aim is to reduce morbidity and mortality due to ethnicity-related conditions such as sickle cell disease, cystic fibrosis and thalassaemia. Data from the GP practices is used to gain details of the morbidity and mortality of the population in relation to ethnicity (comparative need). In addition focus groups are conducted to obtain the views of representatives of each ethnic group regarding their health needs and service provision (felt and expressed need). In the light of the findings, a cost-benefit analysis is undertaken to identify the changes in service provision that would benefit the whole population in terms of reduction in morbidity and mortality. An action plan is developed and presented to representatives of the various ethnic groups (requirement to action). Once agreed, the action plan is implemented and monitored at agreed intervals. A year later data suggest that the health status of the different ethnic groups has improved and the services are embedded permanently in the provision for the local population. The next priority for the PCT is to reduce the number of working days lost to mental health problems in the local community and this becomes the focus of an HNA.

CONCLUSION

An important factor to consider in undertaking an HNA is the ethical implications. Consider this example. A community specialist practitioner is concerned about the health of the local traveller population and wants to carry out an HNA. She has been told that there will be no additional resources to help them even if she finds they do have specific health needs. She feel that funds could be diverted from a local and very popular women's health group as the majority of those who attend seem to have no health problems and just go for coffee and a chat. This raises ethical questions such as:

- Should an HNA be undertaken in relation to a specific client group or in relation to the total population?
- Should HNAs include a cost-benefit analysis?
- Should HNAs concern itself with allocation of resources?

Whilst it is beyond the scope of this chapter to address these questions in detail, it is important to recognise that HNA does carry ethical implications that need to be considered.

FURTHER READING

Hawtin, M. and Percy-Smith, J. (2007) *Community Profiling: A Practical Guide*, 2nd edn. Buckingham: Open University Press.
Hooper, J. and Longworth, P. (2002) *Health Needs Assessment Workbook*. London: Health Development Agency.

22 Planning Public Health Initiatives

Janine Talley

DEFINITION

Whilst there is no generally accepted definition of planning (Lenihan, 2005), planning is commonly used to describe decision-making processes including elements such as setting goals, developing strategies, and outlining the tasks and schedules involved in accomplishing the goals. In the context of public health the goals are related to making things happen that will support the health and wellbeing of populations. Planning elements and processes may be explicit or may be implicit and be associated with terms such as policy, programme, strategy, operational, priority, aim, objective, long-term, action, work, business (Naidoo and Wills, 2000; Health Communication Unit, 2007). Planning has value both as a process and as a route to outcomes including strategic and operational guidance on how to reach public health improvement objectives. Planning may be proactive, responsive or reactive (Nutbeam, 1996), formal or informal and form part of any size of initiative.

KEY POINTS

Planning public health initiatives:

- is important for reasons of effectiveness and accountability;
- may be a form of rational decision-making;
- may require different ways of thinking in complex situations.

DISCUSSION

Planning is an increasingly important and challenging aspect of public health activity and is necessary to ensure effective outcomes, make best use of limited resources and provide accountability. Planning supports management of existing and anticipated threats to public health (coronary heart disease, depression, obesity), as well as extreme and unexpected situations (natural disasters, terrorism, pandemics).

Plans address what you are trying to achieve, what you are going to do and how you will know if it has been successful (Ewles and Simnett, 2003). Public health planning has traditionally been approached as a form of rational decision-making (Lenihan, 2005) – a series of decisions, from general and strategic decisions to specific operational details, based on the gathering and analysis of a wide range of information (Health Communication Unit, 2007). Essentially a problem, need or priority is defined, possible solutions are proposed, the best course of action is decided on the basis of a range of factors including evidence and resources, the action is implemented and processes and outcomes are monitored and evaluated.

Elements which should/could be part of public health planning include:

- underpinning purpose, values, paradigms, theories;
- understanding of context (social, political, cultural, policy, economic, environmental, geographical etc.);
- collaborative working;
- meaningful participation of key stakeholders (including individuals and communities);
- needs;
- resources (human and financial);
- evidence to inform all stages of the process (quantitative and qualitative);
- evaluation.

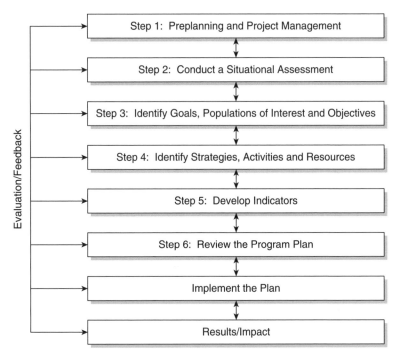

Figure 22.1 *Health Promotion Project Planning: Overview*

*A true copy of this Figure can be found at http://www.thcu.ca/infoandresources/
publications/Planning.wkbk.content.apr01.format.oct06.pdf*

Models have been developed to describe and inform planning of public
health initiatives (see Tones and Green, 2004; Lenihan, 2005; Earle
et al., 2007; Health Communication Unit, 2007). Examples include the
Precede–Proceed Model (Green and Kreuter, 1999) and the THCU
six-step approach (Health Communication Unit, 2007) which is shown
in Figure 22.1.

The model incorporates many of the key elements listed above.
Within the UK context situational assessment would recognise priorities such as reducing health inequalities and increasing community
participation. Higher priority is being given to evidence-based
approaches and the need for practitioners to develop an understanding of evidence sources, research methodologies, principles of interpretation and application to practice. HM Treasury (2004) highlighted
general lack of 'evidence about the cost-effectiveness of public health

and preventative policies or their practical implementation'. The National Institute for Health and Clinical Excellence (NICE, www.nice.org.uk) Centre for Public Health Excellence and other bodies such as Health England and the National Public Health Library are contributing to the development of a more robust evidence base on the clinical and cost-effectiveness of public health interventions. The nature of the evidence and the way in which it is used will vary according to the nature of the intervention. So for example, a community initiative may give greater weighting to evidence of expressed need than to epidemiological evidence.

Planning public health initiatives may be impaired by factors such as differing views on priorities and goals, assumptions, a weak evidence base, short time scales, inadequate resources or political agendas. Planning is value laden with political, ethical and moral dimensions. In practice it may be piecemeal, incremental, *ad hoc*. Flexibility and an approach based on incremental small steps rather than grand plans can be necessary and more appropriate in some circumstances.

In line with wider changes in how we think about the way the world works, new ideas are emerging to inform and shape public health planning. The field of complexity science challenges assumptions about an orderly, predictable, simple, cause and effect world and the applicability of rational planning. Many threats to public health are complex and multi-factorial, e.g. coronary heart disease and obesity. A complexity approach uses ecological metaphors based on relational thinking where individuals and organisations can be seen as complex adaptive systems. Decision-making is based on working with the properties of systems, facilitating adaptation to changing contexts and strengthening self-organising forces. Opportunities where conditions are ripe for natural success are sought, and knowledge can be built up and applied without advance knowledge of what actions will be needed. The matrix in Figure 22.2 (Stacey, 2002) is helpful in looking at decision-making in relation to dimensions of certainty and agreement.

Where we are close to certainty, cause and effect links are clear and there is evidence and experience available to extrapolate outcomes with reasonable certainty. Where we are far from certainty, causal links are unclear and the situation may be unfamiliar, with little experience and evidence to draw on. The agreement axis relates to the level of agreement between individuals or groups in relation to an issue or decision. The model suggests:

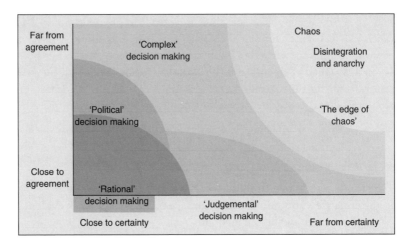

Figure 22.2 *Stacey matrix*

(Legible version of diagram available here: http://www.gp-training.net/training/ consultation/ equipoise/complexity.htm)

- Rational decision-making where we are close to both certainty and agreement. So we follow the process of gathering evidence and information to inform paths of action aimed at achieving anticipated outcomes.
- Political decision-making where we have a great deal of certainty but low levels of agreement on outcomes and rational planning would not work. This prioritises activities such as building collaborations and coalitions and processes of negotiation, and compromise.
- Judgemental decision-making where agreement is high but certainty is low. The focus of planning here is on making progress towards an agreed future situation although it is not possible to predetermine the way to get there.

In the zone of complexity (edge of chaos) there are high levels of creativity, innovation, and breaking with the past to create new modes of operating. A diversity of approaches is needed to deal with diversity of contexts. Ways of knowing outside the scientific and rational inform progress. Cooper and Geyer (2007) provide a good introduction to complexity and its application to planning diabetes care.

For strategic planning where the future is unpredictable, techniques such as horizon scanning and scenario planning (Neiner et al., 2004) can be useful. Scenario planning involves imagining plausible futures, creating adaptive strategies, sensing emerging direction, and building on what works.

CASE STUDY: PRIMARY SCHOOL INITIATIVE TO PREVENT RISK FACTORS FOR OBESITY (BASED ON SAHOTA ET AL., 2001)

A school-based programme was planned to prevent risk factors for obesity. Planning was informed by published evidence on the prevalence and health impact of obesity and was in line with national targets for obesity reduction. An intervention programme of established effectiveness was used – The Active Programme Promoting Lifestyle Education in School (APPLES). The approach was multidisciplinary and multi-agency and population based. The programme team included a dietician (project manager), a community paediatrician, a health promotion specialist, a psychologist, an obesity physician and a nutritional epidemiologist. It was underpinned by the Health Promoting Schools philosophy which looks both at the whole school and the context in which it is set, so school, family and community were involved, with a whole school approach addressing ethos, policies, management style and attitudes of staff. To ensure ownership and successful implementation, schools, teachers, parents, caterers and pupils participated in the development of the programme. The initiative was based on school action plans, developed by individual schools on the basis of their views and perceived needs. Interventions included teacher training, modification of school meals, and the development of school action plans which targeted the curriculum, physical education, tuck shops and playground activities. These aimed to influence dietary and physical activity behaviour as well as knowledge. Monitoring of progress towards targets was included in the form of regular staff meetings and surveys of packed lunches, break time snacks and playground activities. Systematic evaluation was included. Outcome measures included response rates to questionnaires, teachers' evaluation of training and input, success of school action plans, content of school meals, body mass index, diet, physical activity, psychological state, and children's knowledge of healthy living and self-reported behaviour. Methodology for needs assessment and evaluation included questionnaires and focus groups.

CONCLUSION

Planning, whether formal or informal is a key element of any initiative aimed at improving public health. Planning should take into account a wide range of factors, and best practice indicates making central the needs of those to whom initiatives are directed and an evidence based approach. A range of planning models are available which can provide useful support for practice. However, rational approaches need to be considered carefully in relation to real contexts which are often complex and unpredictable. New approaches based on complexity science are offering different perspectives on context and approaches to planning in public health.

FURTHER READING

Tones, K. and Green, J. (2004) *Health Promotion: Planning Strategies*. London: Sage.
World Health Organization (2003) *Fourth futures forum on high-level decision-makers' tools for decision making in public health* [online]. Retrieved 25 January 2008, from http://www.euro.who.int/document/e80895.pdf

23 Evaluating Public Health Programmes

Elaine Hogard

DEFINITION

In its broadest sense evaluation means determining the value of something or someone. It is a constant human activity to make judgements on how good or bad we find people, things and ideas. In that sense anything can be evaluated and, arguably, our view of the social and physical world is permeated with evaluations of people, things, ideas, events and institutions. Indeed theorists have argued that our identity and self is determined, in large part, by the ways in which we identify with and

key concepts in public health

place value on entities in the social and physical world (Weinreich and Saunderson, 2003).

In a more specific sense evaluation refers to the activities of professional evaluators who apply their techniques to making judgements about the effectiveness of programmes and initiatives usually, but not exclusively, in the public sector. Some of the main focuses for such evaluations are programmes in education, social care, healthcare, community safety and regional development. They of course include evaluations of various initiatives and programmes aimed at improving public health.

Typically programme evaluations aim to determine whether the stated objectives of a programme have been met. They may also be concerned with establishing how they have been met and whether the objectives of the programme have been met cost-effectively. Evaluations often try to find out how various stakeholders, including recipients and providers, have viewed the programme and how they would describe its strengths and weaknesses.

These concerns with outcomes, processes and stakeholder perspectives have led us to propose an Evaluation trident which suggests that all evaluations address three main questions: did the programme achieve its stated objectives? What was the process by which the programme was delivered and how did this impact on the objectives? And what did the various stakeholders involved think of the programme? (Ellis and Hogard, 2006; see Figure 23.1)

KEY POINTS

Evaluators:

- gather data to answer evaluation questions;
- use the full range of social science methods to gather data;
- draw conclusions from the data.

Evaluation:

- is usually carried out by an independent and objective third party;
- demonstrates public accountability for the programme providers and funders;
- can contribute feedback to improve the delivery of the programme both formatively and summatively;

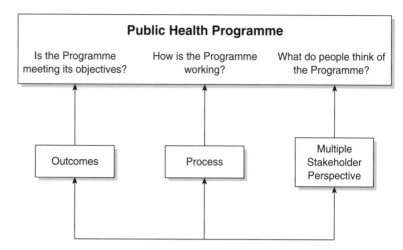

Figure 23.1 *The Evaluation Trident (Ellis and Hogard, 2006)*

- addresses a number of research reports;
- can recommend future action;
- reports can help to profile and publicise the programme.

DISCUSSION

Much work in public health consists of programmes that are aimed at improving the health status of individuals and groups through changing attitudes and behaviour. There is a strong imperative to evaluate such programmes for a number of reasons. First there is a need to demonstrate public accountability for the investment that has been made in the programme. Such accountability should go beyond the assurances of providers that all is going well. An external and objective view should be formed on whether the programme is meeting its objectives and doing so in a cost-effective fashion. Secondly the evaluation should provide feedback to the providers so that they can develop and improve their delivery. Thirdly the evaluation should ensure that lessons are learned from the programme to inform future programmes. Fourthly the evaluation may unearth new knowledge regarding programme delivery and its effect on outcomes. Fifthly the evaluation report will profile and publicise the programme and disseminate good

practice and may lead to other forms of publication: academic, professional and popular.

The first job of the evaluator is to agree with the providers and the
funders the objectives of the programme and crucially the evidence that
will be taken as indicative that the objectives have been met. This part
of the evaluation is often problematic since objectives may have been
expressed in general rather than specific terms and they may not easily
translate into measurable outcomes. Having agreed objectives and outcome measures it will be the job of the evaluator to ensure that evidence is available regarding the extent to which they have been met.

The second job for the evaluator is to establish exactly what the programme is, who is involved, what they do, and what the recipients get
from the programme. This part of the evaluation is concerned with the
processes of the programme. These processes must be described in
detail, to allow for the programme to be replicated and to allow connections to be made between what happens in the programme and what
is achieved through these happenings. So if a programme includes
processes of education, as many public health programmes do, what is
the effect and impact of these educational processes on recipients? How
have their attitudes and behaviours changed? How do these changes
reflect the stated objectives and outcomes of the programme?

Evaluators may attempt to tease out the theoretical assumptions that
drive the programme. What assumptions do the providers have regarding
the relationship between the processes they carry out and the desired outcomes? Data from the evaluation should allow the theory, which may be
relatively implicit, to be tested. Knowledge of the process in detail allows
for it to be costed and these costs related to the effects in terms of outcomes and impact. This equation allows for a cost-effectiveness analysis,
particularly if comparisons can be made with other methods and costs to
achieve the same outcomes.

The evaluators should ensure that there are opportunities for all
stakeholders to articulate their views of the programme. The evaluation
should aim to include multiple stakeholder perspectives, including not
only recipients and providers but others affected by or involved in the
delivery of the programme.

The methods used by evaluators to answer their questions regarding
output, process, viewpoints and causality draw upon the full repertoire
of data-gathering techniques in the social and behavioural sciences.
They will include both qualitative and quantitative methods and most

evaluations could be described as mixed method. They will include such techniques as observation, interviews, focus groups, questionnaires, process recording and documentary analysis. The common thread is that the methods will be used to answer evaluation questions of the kind outlined above.

Ideally an evaluation should be carried out in partnership with the programme providers in that they should appreciate the advantages of externality. The evaluators should demonstrate a familiarity with and sympathy with the approach of the programme.

Given the limitations of funding and available resources, evaluations will usually focus on a number of small projects each contributing to the overall evaluation but concentrating on the issues agreed to be salient by the evaluators and programme providers. The information produced through these projects can contribute to the refinement and development of the programme during the life of the evaluation.

The final report will be a summation of these projects and provide an overview of the extent to which the programme has met its objectives, the key features of the process and their effectiveness, and the views of all involved. The report will conclude with recommendations which will ensure that lessons are learned for future programme delivery.

CASE STUDY

The trident method has proved itself in more than 50 contracted evaluations. The evaluation of a Sure Start scheme provides a good example. The first question was to establish the objectives or outcomes that the scheme was intended to meet and the evidence available of their accomplishment. Two kinds of objective were found. First the Sure Start Scheme, like all such schemes, was intended to meet objectives set by the government as a condition of funding. There were 23 objectives and the scheme was obliged to gather evidence and report on their success annually. A typical objective was to increase breast-feeding. Statistics were available to demonstrate that this had been achieved but it was difficult to claim that the activities of a single scheme were the sole or even primary cause. A second level of outcomes was set by the scheme itself and included, for example, the number of parents/carers who turned up to the programme. However, such local objectives were concerned more with process than with actual outcomes, most of which were longer term than the scheme itself.

The second prong of the trident addressed the processes of the Sure Start scheme and data were gathered on the organisation and management of the scheme and the activities that the scheme promoted including, for example, mother and toddler music sessions. These descriptions of process allowed for replication could, in principle, be related to the achievement of particular objectives although this proved difficult in practice. Finally the key stakeholders in the scheme were identified: these included the parents and carers, Sure Start staff, volunteers, and related professionals. The views of these stakeholders were solicited using interviews, focus groups and questionnaires. Whilst the predominant flavour of these views was positive, valuable insights were gained into features that could be improved. One interesting development was the involvement of volunteers in the design of a questionnaire and this found, for example, that those put off from attending Sure Start sessions had identified them with social services with which they had had negative experiences.

CONCLUSION

Evaluation is pervasive in the public sector, including the key area of public health. Evaluators should ensure that key questions are asked regarding outcomes, processes and stakeholder views and that data are gathered to answer these questions in a scientific and rigorous fashion. The evaluation should contribute to the improvement of the programme both within the life of the evaluation and subsequently. Evaluation should, therefore, link strategic issues and policy formulation with operational issues and lessons learned.

FURTHER READING

Chen, H.T. (2005) *Practical Program Evaluation*. London: Sage.
Shaw, I.F., Greene, J.C. and Mark, M.M. (eds) (2006) *The Sage Handbook of Evaluation*. London: Sage.

evaluating public health programmes

24 Health Impact Assessment

Rachel A. Wells

DEFINITION

Health impact assessment (HIA) is defined as an assessment of the effects that an action or group of actions may have on the health of a population. The population may be defined in the broadest sense and may be geographical or a community of interest. Scott-Samuel defined HIA as 'the estimation of the effects of a specified action on the health of a defined population' (Scott-Samuel, 1998).

The WHO definition is 'a combination of procedures, methods and tools by which a policy, programme or project may be judged as to its potential effects on the health of a population, and the distribution of those effects within the population' (WHO, 1999).

KEY POINTS

- democracy – the involvement of a wide range of stakeholders;
- equity – assessment of impacts from a wide range of angles but with a focus on the most vulnerable groups for whom the impacts may be more significant;
- sustainable development – the short- and long-term perspective and ethical use of evidence (WHO, 2007). All of these have resonance with public health professionals as also important to much good public health practice.

DISCUSSION

The use of HIA can therefore be wide ranging and extend to multi-faceted developments such as perhaps the new Wembley Stadium in London or relate to much smaller developments – small new housing developments, the moving of a school, or other actions which may impact on a local community. HIA can also be applied to regeneration initiatives and other policy decisions – provision of youth and community service for example at local level or the development of a city-wide policy on waste management. Much has been written on some of the specifics of HIA in a regeneration context, for example. This might be in regard to the provision of new services, or changing the delivery or location of existing services.

Policy context

In England the Department of Health is supportive of HIA as an assessment tool and as part of the White Paper *Choosing Health* (DH, 2004b), the government gave a commitment to build health into all future legislation by including health as a component in regulatory impact assessment (RIA). This has since been revised by the Cabinet Office to become impact assessment (IA) and HIA is one of the specific tests within this.

Ideally HIA should be applied before the action to be assessed starts – prospectively. This is not always possible, so the HIA may run at the same time or even be done retrospectively.

The process

There are several models which describe the HIA process, and no one agreed way of undertaking an HIA, though many of the components are of a similar nature (Scott-Samuel et al., 2001 – Impact guidelines).

One of the simplest descriptions is provided by the WHO principles of HIA. The WHO identifies five simple steps:

- Screening
- Scoping
- Appraisal
- Reporting
- Monitoring

Screening

This determines whether it is appropriate to undertake an HIA in the first place. The Impact guidelines suggest a process which identifies four areas to consider in the screening stage: economic issues, outcome issues, epidemiological issues and strategic issues.

Each should be considered with a view to the likely impact of the proposal to give a considered perspective on the need for the HIA process to be taken further (WHO, 1999; Scott-Samuel et al., 2001). Each element is considered and the potential impact identified alongside the groups most likely to be affected. The ranking of elements (proposed by the Impact Guidelines) are particularly useful in crystallising the focus on the screening and helping to form a perspective on the important elements to consider. At this point the intended focus sometimes shifts, as elements to be included in the HIA emerge as more important than first thought.

Scott-Samuel et al. (2001) propose that before any recommendation is made it is useful to work through each of the four elements.

Scoping

One of the key activities of this stage is the establishment of a steering group to oversee the HIA. This group would negotiate the terms of reference and set the scope of the HIA, determining the boundaries – i.e. what the HIA will cover and what will be excluded – and the methodology for the next step. The outcomes of the scoping would be used to inform this.

Appraisal

This is where the HIA gathers pace as this stage usually involves the collection of information from a range of sources and the use of a range of methods to cover all the issues that are raised. This might include desktop research in addition to interviews with stakeholders or communities who may be affected by the proposal being assessed. The ranking of information is often carried out and an assessment made with regard to its impact – negative or positive. Workshops are often a key feature of this stage and many include this as a main vehicle for information collection. It is easy to consider this stage to be the most important and though it's true that it provides much of the detailed information, the effectiveness of the appraisal is informed by the screening and the scoping. The workshops are an important way of developing and building views and opinions for this stage of the HIA.

Reporting

At this stage the findings of the appraisal are presented. This is characterised by either excitement or frustration, depending on how the decision-makers interpret and act on your findings.

Monitoring and evaluation

The WHO (1999) suggests that it is important to monitor whether the HIA has worked or not, and good practice would agree. It is important to build in ways to demonstrate whether the process or outcomes of the HIA influence the steps taken by policy-makers/planners who consider the impact of the HIA on furthering the action assessed in the first place. As with all evaluation activities, planning must be scheduled for this at the beginning of the process.

CASE STUDY

There are many example of HIAs available which can provide background information on the wide range of ways in which HIA can be applied. The development of Manchester Airport and redevelopment of Wembley Stadium are good examples of large-scale HIAs.

Redevelopment of Wembley, north London

The HIA of the redevelopment of Wembley encompassed a wide range of proposals, including the new National Stadium, around 4,000 new homes, commercial and retail developments and leisure opportunities. In addition to this, changes in the transport infrastructure were required. It was recognised by the local planning authorities that the new developments were likely to have significant impacts on the local population and the HIA was initiated to make an independent assessment of the plans before formal applications were made (Barnes et al., 2004).

The stages of the HIA reflect the Impact Guidelines in the establishment of a group to lead the HIA review of data sources for background purposes, collection of data through workshops, and analysis of the information gathered. There was a further review of additional evidence to support and qualify the workshop findings and finally the presentation of the result to the local strategy group. The HIA was part of a number of initiatives in Brent Primary Care Trust that determined local needs and developed responses to health inequalities in the borough.

The key issues, for the HIA, were identified through discussion in rapid HIA workshops with a range of attendees from the locality or representing it. The results of this were that social and community cohesion, quality of life and opportunities for local people ranked highly, along with transport, employment (and unemployment), as likely to be influenced most significantly by the Wembley proposals. Housing and leisure were important to those taking part, with health and social care, education, environmental concerns and crime featuring less. A number of specific population groups were also identified, by the process, for which some factors were likely to be more significant: this included people moving to the area for work, to visit, groups with particular needs, children and young people, older people, people from minority ethnic groups – both long-standing and new arrivals.

The HIA addressed each of the issues identified in turn to consider the evidence from routine health and other data sources to inform the discussion on the issues raised. This was brought together with the development plans to give a full picture of the potential health impacts – both beneficial and negative – of the proposed development, taking into account the construction phase as a key element (as far as could be estimated). Recommendations for each issue followed in a separate section of the report, which was then taken to the commissioners of the HIA for consideration and for decision (Barnes et al., 2004).

CONCLUSION

HIAs often constrained by costs and time. There are numerous instances when an HIA has been put into the planning process for a development or consultation but this hasn't taken place due to time running out or the finance just not being there. Sometimes you will find that HIAs are watered down to a considerable extent so that their value is questionable as a way of informing decision-makers of the impacts of a policy or development. However, one of the key benefits of HIA is that it provides a systematic approach to the collection and recording of information from a wide range of sources.

FURTHER READING

Scott-Samuel, A., Birley, M. and Ardern, K. (2001) *The Merseyside Guidelines for Health Impact Assessment*, 2nd edn. London: International Health Impact Assessment Consortium.

WHO (1999) *Gothenburg Consensus Paper. Health Impact Assessment: Main Concepts and Suggested Approach*. Brussels: European Centre for Health Policy, WHO Regional Office for Europe.

key concepts in public health

25 Health Protection

Nicholas Fulton Phin

DEFINITION

Within the United Kingdom, there is no clear consensus on the definition of health protection. The Faculty of Public Health, in describing public health practice, identifies three overlapping domains:

- health improvement/promotion;
- improving health services;
- health protection.

The five topics included in the health protection domain are listed as:

- infectious diseases;
- chemicals and poisons;
- radiation;
- emergency response;
- environmental health hazards.

This chapter uses a definition of health protection adapted from *Getting Ahead of the Curve: A Strategy for Combating Infectious Diseases* (DH, 2002), in which the establishment of the Health Protection Agency was proposed. In this document, the Chief Medical Officer for England acknowledged that infectious diseases are only one of the threats to human health and that there are other threats from the physical environment such as chemical and radiation incidents. Health protection can therefore be simply defined as: 'the prevention or mitigation of threats to human health from the external environment including infectious diseases, chemicals and radiation'.

- Health protection is part of public health practice, which focuses on preventing or mitigating all hazards to human health from the external environment.
- Health protection is the province of a number of organisations at local and national level working together to protect the public health.
- The Health Protection Agency is a source of expert advice and knowledge on infectious diseases, chemicals and radiation but does not have executive responsibility for health protection.

DISCUSSION

The term health protection is very broad and overlaps with other aspects of public health. There is therefore potential for confusion between health promotion/improvement and health protection, given that the ultimate outcome of both approaches is improved health. It is perhaps more helpful to consider health protection as those actions that are taken to protect individuals or the population from factors in the external environment, and health promotion as those things that people choose to do to protect themselves. Food is a good example; health protection is about ensuring that the food that is eaten is safe and free from infection or toxins; health promotion is about eating the right types of food in the right proportions to ensure that nutrition is optimised and body mass index is within a healthy range.

It is also important to understand that health protection is the responsibility of many organisations. Although there is a national organisation called the Health Protection Agency, its functions are essentially the provision of expert advice and information. The executive functions associated with health protection, treatment, prosecution, prohibition and enforcement are discharged by organisations as diverse as local authorities, NHS Primary Care Trusts, the Health and Safety Executive and the Food Standards Agency.

In response to the growing need for a strong, integrated and modern system of healthy protection to respond not just to infectious diseases but to other external threats, such as winter floods, climate change, the World Trade Center attack and the deliberate release of anthrax in the US, a review of the existing health protection systems was undertaken. In the report *Getting Ahead of the Curve* (DH, 2002), produced by the

Chief Medical Officer for England, it was recommended that a new National Infection and Health Protection Agency should be established. This agency, later shortened to the Health Protection Agency (HPA), would bring together the local aspects of the health protection function within Primary Care Trusts, the Public Health Laboratory Service, the National Radiological Protection Board, the National Focus for Chemical Incidents, and the National Centre for Applied Microbiology and Research.

In bringing all these diverse autonomous organisations together, it was intended that the main functions of this new organisation would be:

- to provide information, expertise and advice on infectious diseases, chemical and radiation hazards;
- to co-ordinate surveillance systems for the prevention and control of infectious diseases in England;
- to develop systems of surveillance to protect against the risks from chemical and radiation hazards;
- to work with the Commission for Health to improve standards of infection control in hospitals, primary care and other health service premises;
- to assist the NHS and local authorities in investigating and managing outbreaks of infectious disease, and chemical and radiation incidents;
- to advise on national and local policy in relation to the prevention and control of infectious disease and protection from chemical and radiation hazards.

The HPA came into being in 2003 initially as a special authority of the NHS but in 2005 it became established as an 'arm's length body' by the Health Protection Agency Act 2004. The agency is structured into a number of divisions providing advice and expertise on a range of subjects. These are:

- *The Centre for Infections* – this provides national infectious disease surveillance, specialist and reference microbiology, the co-ordination and investigation of national and uncommon outbreaks and advice to central government on policy, and it responds to international health alerts.
- *The Centre for Radiation, Chemical Hazards and Environmental Hazards* – this division advises on ionising and non-ionising radiation, including laboratory and technical services, advises central government on the human health effects from chemicals in the soil, water and waste, and provides support and advice to the NHS on toxicology.

- *The Centre for Emergency Preparedness and Response* – this has an important role in preparing for and co-ordinating responses to potential healthcare emergencies, including acts of deliberate release. It also has a major role in running training courses and emergency exercises to test plans and preparedness.
- *Local and Regional Services* – this is the largest of the divisions and works alongside the NHS and local authorities to provide specialist support in infection control, communicable disease and emergency planning.
- *The Regional Microbiology Network* – this provides frontline diagnostic and microbiological services to the NHS and local health protection units. The network also manages the food, water and environmental laboratories that do so much of the analysis of suspected foodstuffs and materials.

The case history below gives an example of how an incident would be managed across the agency. A communicable disease example has been chosen because the issues relating to the response to a chemical and radiation incident are dealt with in chapter 31.

CASE HISTORY

A large supermarket, because of a shortage of vegetables for its salads, switches from a UK supplier to one abroad. Unknown to the supermarket and the supplier, the water used to irrigate the crops has become contaminated with faecal material. Certain components in the salad now contain low levels of an unusual salmonella – salmonella Boratz. The salad product is distributed mainly to supermarkets in the north of England but some is also supplied to shops in the south-west.

Over the course of a few days, some customers eating the salad become unwell with diarrhoea and stomach pains. Some of those affected with symptoms become ill enough to visit their GP where, in some instances, faecal samples are taken for microbiological investigation; others are sent home with 'gastric flu'.

In the laboratories where the samples have been sent, a salmonella with an unusual serotype is identified. The local health protection units of the patients are alerted, the patients' GPs are sent the results, and isolates of the salmonella are sent to the reference laboratory at the HPA Centre for Infections for further classification.

The consultant in communicable disease control (CCDC) in the HPU informs the environmental health officers (EHOs) of the local authority where the case is resident and they arrange to visit the patient to get details of the illness, occupation, travel abroad, information on other cases, and a food history prior to the illness. At the same time, the CCDC receives a formal notification from the GP.

After a few days, the Centre for Infection identifies the salmonella as Boratz, a salmonella seen in very small numbers in the UK and usually identified only in travellers from abroad.

The numbers of isolations of salmonella Boratz start to increase and breach national exceedance levels. It is becoming clear that these cases are clustered in the north. A national teleconference involving the CCDCs with cases, the regional epidemiologists from affected regions, and the epidemiologists at the Centre for Infections is convened. It is agreed that this is an outbreak and there is an early indication in the completed food questionnaires that consumption of salad may be implicated. It is decided that a case control study with a more detailed questionnaire, a trawling questionnaire, would be needed for past and future cases. In addition, samples of any salad from cases would be helpful. Further genetic analyses of the strains will also be undertaken to establish that these were linked.

The local HPUs and local authorities administered questionnaires to controls and cases and the EHOs were able to obtain samples of salad: these were sent to the HPA food and water laboratories for analysis. Salmonella was identified from the salad supplied by the supermarket and this was corroborated by the results from the case control study. The Food Standards Agency (FSA) was informed and investigations between the FSA and local EHOs focused on the factory where the salad was prepared. The FSA convinced the company that they should voluntarily withdraw the product from the shops. Further investigations linked the infected salad to a supplier abroad. The relevant authorities in that country were notified.

FURTHER READING

Department of Health (2002) *Getting Ahead of the Curve: A Strategy for Combating Infectious Diseases*. London: Department of Health.

Department of Health (2005) *Health Protection in the 21st Century: Understanding the Burden of Disease*. London: Department of Health.

26 Immunisation

Michelle Falconer

DEFINITION

Infectious diseases remain one of the biggest causes of death in humans and over 3 million children die every year from diseases that are preventable. Immunisation is described by the Health Protection Agency (HPA) as 'the process of protecting individuals from infection through passive or active immunity'.

Active immunity occurs when the immune system produces antibodies against a specific antigen (a molecule which is recognised by the immune system and induces an immune response, e.g. a virus or bacterium) (Galazka, 1993). This can follow immunisation or natural disease and protection for the individual is usually lifelong. Passive immunity requires the administration of antibodies directly to the individual; protection from passive immunity is of short duration and immunisation is typically used to protect an individual from infection when rapid protection is required.

The immune system responds to millions of specific antigens daily (Salisbury et al., 2006), and the aim of immunisation is to produce a rapid, protective immune response upon re-exposure of the individual to the antigen contained in the vaccine (Griffin et al., 2003). Although it may take several weeks for immunity to develop following immunisation, the process induces a primary adaptive immune response which establishes immunological memory in the individual. If the individual is re-exposed to the same antigen, a secondary response occurs. This secondary response occurs very rapidly and the antibodies produced are highly specific, though booster doses of some vaccines are required to sustain the duration of immunological memory (Helbert, 2006).

KEY POINTS

- Immunisation is the process used to deliver an immunogenic substance to stimulate an immune response which will protect against infectious disease.

- Vaccines may be live (attenuated) or inactivated and work by inducing active immunity and providing immunological memory.
- The primary aim of immunisation is to protect the individual who receives the vaccine.
- Individuals who cannot be immunised will also benefit from routine immunisation programmes through herd immunity.
- Most individuals can be immunised with all vaccines and there are very few individuals for whom immunisation is contra-indicated.

DISCUSSION

Immunisation is one of the safest and most cost-effective interventions that we have available (Salisbury et al., 2006), and there is no doubt that it has had a significant impact on public health: immunisation to protect against smallpox led to the eradication of the disease in 1980, which is thought to have prevented 350 million new cases and around 40 million deaths. Other infectious diseases such as polio and measles are being targeted by the World Health Organization for eradication in the future.

The overall aims of immunisation have been described as being:

- to protect the individual and communities from infectious diseases and their associated mortality, morbidity and long-term sequelae;
- to prevent and contain outbreaks of disease;
- to eradicate infectious diseases (UK Guidance on best practice in vaccine administration, DH, 2001d).

In the UK, public health interventions such as improved sanitation have ensured the availability of clean drinking water and the efficient and hygienic disposal of sewage; however, the provision of an effective immunisation programme is essential to protect individuals and communities against diseases that cannot be controlled through hygiene measures alone. Although sanitary changes have impacted on the incidence of diseases such as cholera and typhoid, it is recognised that such changes are ineffective against diseases that are not transmitted via the faeco-oral route.

For example, influenza is a highly infectious disease that is transmitted by direct contact with the respiratory secretions of an infected person and good respiratory hygiene is essential to control the infection. HIV and hepatitis B are blood-borne viruses. Both would require a change in personal and/or sexual behaviour to prevent transmission or acquisition of the virus.

immunisation

Population increases are impacting on the incidence of some infectious diseases. One example is Lyme disease which is becoming more common in the UK as people move to areas that were previously forested or take part in outdoor activities in such areas.

Travel outside the UK also brings with it the possibility of exposure to infections that individuals would not necessarily be at risk from in the UK such as tick-borne encephalitis and Japanese encephalitis, and in some countries evidence of immunisation is compulsory: for example a yellow fever certificate is required for entry into certain countries when travelling from endemic areas.

Finally, immunisation against certain infections may be a requirement of some occupations. This may include rabies vaccine for bat handlers, and healthcare workers may require immunisation against hepatitis B, measles, mumps, rubella, tuberculosis, influenza and varicella. This will usually be determined following an occupational health assessment.

Vaccine composition

Vaccines may be live attenuated (weakened), inactivated, toxoid or sub-unit and the antigenic component may consist of toxins, bacteria or viruses, surface proteins or fragments of the cell wall or capsule of the organism. Additionally, vaccines may contain adjuvants such as aluminium salts to enhance the immune response; stabilisers to maintain the potency of the vaccine and to protect it from adverse conditions and residuals from the manufacturing process such as antibiotics, egg or yeast proteins. Vaccines should provide optimum immunological protection with minimal trauma for the individual and several criteria for an ideal vaccine have been identified (Janeway et al., 2005).

The vaccine should:

- be safe and effective;
- provide sustained protection for the individual from the disease against which it is designed to protect;
- be cost-effective;
- be acceptable to the recipients.

If an immunisation programme is effective it can also protect unvaccinated members of the community if herd immunity is achieved. This occurs when a large proportion of the population has been immunised and means it is less likely that individuals who remain susceptible will come into contact with infected persons.

Although vaccines are very effective at protecting against disease, vaccine failures do sometimes occur. Primary vaccine failure occurs when an individual fails to respond to a vaccine, and secondary vaccine failure occurs when protection initially obtained from a vaccine wanes over time.

The UK childhood immunisation programme

Many factors are taken into account when deciding on national immunisation policy (Salisbury et al., 2002). Mathematical modelling may be used to predict disease patterns, the impact of different vaccination options and the economic consequences of any changes to the immunisation programme. Additionally, the safety and efficacy of the vaccine, the epidemiology of the disease and public attitudes to the disease and the vaccine need to be considered.

Currently, the routine UK childhood immunisation programme protects children against 10 vaccine-preventable diseases (Salisbury et al., 2006). However, the programme continues to evolve and changes to it may occur as new vaccines are developed. Following a recommendation by the Joint Committee on Vaccination and Immunisation (JCVI) the Department of Health has announced that a vaccine to protect against human papilloma virus will be added to the childhood immunisation programme in 2008. The principal aim of this is to protect girls against future risk of cervical cancer.

CASE STUDY

Surveillance of vaccine preventable diseases and uptake of vaccines is undertaken for all vaccines offered as part of the UK childhood programme. This enables identification of trends, calculation of vaccine coverage, estimates of vaccine efficacy and modifications to the immunisation programme to be made.

The impact of immunisation on Hib epidemiology

Haemophilus Influenzae type b (Hib) spreads through close contact with an infected person or carrier of the organism and for young children it is the leading cause of childhood meningitis, with a case fatality rate of 4% and up to 11% of those affected having permanent neurological sequelae such as seizures, deafness or intellectual impairment (Salisbury et al., 2006).

Prior to the introduction of an effective Hib vaccine, there were an estimated 445,000 cases of invasive Hib disease in children under the age of 5 years globally, resulting in 115,000 deaths.

The first vaccines to be produced to protect against Hib were not very effective in children under the age of 18 months. However, the immunogenic response to the vaccine was improved when a conjugate vaccine was introduced in the UK during 1992. The conjugate vaccine contains the outer polysaccharide capsule linked to a carrier protein which is recognised by the immune system, enabling a response to the vaccine to be made.

Yearly outbreaks of Hib disease were observed in the UK prior to routine immunisation, but by 1998 there was a 98 per cent reduction in the number of laboratory confirmed cases of Hib in children under the age of 5 years. This brought with it an additional reduction in the circulation of Hib bacteria, resulting in declining disease rates also being observed in adults and unvaccinated older children (PL/CMO/2003/1).

During 2003, a catch-up campaign was undertaken as the enhanced surveillance system identified a gradual increase in the number of cases of Hib disease in children under the age of 4 years.

Continued surveillance has demonstrated that immunity gained from a primary schedule of three doses of Hib vaccine wanes during infancy so a booster dose was added to the childhood programme during 2006. It is expected that the addition of this booster dose will further lower the rates of Hib disease and will also extend the duration of protection against Hib.

CONCLUSION

Immunisation is recognised as being among the safest, most cost-effective and most successful public health interventions available for preventing diseases and the complications that arise from them (Kassianos, 2001).

It is expected that future developments in vaccine manufacturing technology will ensure that immunisation remains at the forefront of public health interventions for preventing disease. Work continues on the development of vaccines to prevent diseases such as malaria, AIDS, salmonella and chlamydia and on the development of therapeutic vaccines to fight rather than prevent diseases such as multiple sclerosis, diabetes and rheumatoid arthritis. New technologies will also bring opportunities to deliver vaccines in new ways and in new combinations (www.abpi.org.uk).

As the UK immunisation programme continues to evolve, it remains essential that all those involved in the delivery of the childhood programme are able to provide up-to-date, evidence-based information to those attending for immunisation.

FURTHER READING

Plotkin, S., Orenstein, W. and Offit, P. (2003) *Vaccines*. Philadelphia: Saunders.
Salisbury, D., Ramsay, M. and Noakes, K. (eds) (2006) *Immunisation against Infectious Disease*. London: The Stationery Office.

27 Public Health and Health Promotion

Frances Wilson

DEFINITION

The 'new' public health includes public health and health promotion, seen as two complementary areas of practice (Naidoo and Wills, 2005). However, their origins are clearly defined, with health promotion emerging during the 1970s and 80s as a force to prevent ill health, differentiating it from the public health purpose of disease prevention. Their relationship and purpose in the twenty-first century may be contentious as health promotion develops as a unique discipline.

The Ottawa Charter (WHO, 1986) established the core principles of health promotion more than 20 years ago. Health promotion is now regarded as a branch of modern public health aimed at tackling the major determinants of health, thus contributing to positive health development. It is applicable to all sectors of society, public, private or voluntary (WHO, 2005).

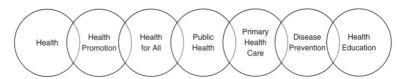

Figure 27.1 *Seven core definitions central to the concept of health promotion, adapted from the* Health Promotion Glossary *(WHO, 1998)*

The *Health Promotion Glossary* (WHO, 1998) is a starting point for students of health promotion and includes seven definitions central to the health promotion concept (Fig. 27.1) along with a compendium of associated terms. An understanding of health, health promotion, health education, public health, and health and wellbeing is essential to current public health and health promotion practices.

A revised glossary (Smith et al., 2006) adds to the list, including burden of disease, capacity building, evidence-based health promotion, global health, health impact assessment, self-efficacy, social marketing, sustainable health promotion actions and wellness.

The following definition, from the Bangkok Charter, gives a new direction to health promotion with emphasis on global health issues: 'Health Promotion works to enable people to increase control over their health and its determinants by developing personal skills, embracing community action, and fostering appropriate public policies, health services and supportive environments. Health Promotion is currently guiding global, national and community health policies, thereby contributing to reducing health risks such as smoking, alcohol consumption, eating habits and physical inactivity' (WHO, 2005). This builds on earlier work such as the Jakarta Declaration (WHO, 1997) and Health 21 (WHO, 1998).

Essential definitions, theories and models of health promotion are discussed in this chapter, along with important WHO milestones and influential UK policies responsible for the advancement of health promotion as a discipline: these are summarised in Figure 27.2.

KEY POINTS

- Health promotion is a branch of modern public health and described as the 'new' public health.
- Health promotion has arguably emerged as a unique discipline with a body of theory and policy that promotes health and wellbeing.

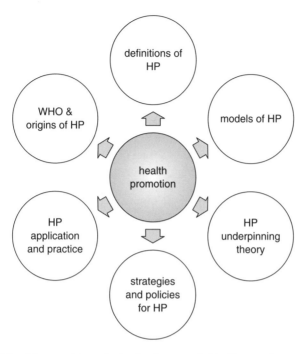

Figure 27.2 *A framework for understanding the concept of health promotion*

- Health promotion strategies are typically associated with broader empowerment based and socio-political approaches.
- Health promotion activities can take place at individual, group, community and organisational levels.
- Models of health promotion can help health promotion specialists describe, analyse, plan and evaluate their activities.

DISCUSSION

The World Health Organization has informed the debate on the development of health promotion as a speciality. Emerging reports build and expand on what has gone before to achieve global engagement and action.

The Lalonde Report (1974) significantly influenced understanding of health and achieving health improvements, being a major departure from the previous emphasis on biomedical interventions. It identified the 'health field concept' within which health could be improved.

Environment and lifestyle offer greater opportunities for promoting public health through behaviour modification, though the emphasis on individual approaches is also a source of criticism (Earle et al., 2007). The importance of environmental influences underpinned the health promotion and 'new' public health movements as healthy public policy developed from this point.

The concept of health and wellbeing which underpins health promotion practice can be interpreted in various ways. One of the earliest definitions of health is: 'Health is a state of complete physical, social and mental wellbeing, not merely the absence of disease or infirmity' (WHO, 1948). This definition of health underpins the Health for All strategy (WHO, 1978) followed by the Declaration of Alma Ata (WHO, 1978b) which focused on the need for accessible primary care systems throughout the world.

The concept was later refined as: 'Health is a resource for everyday life, not the object of living. It is a positive concept emphasising social and personal resources as well as physical capabilities' (WHO, 1986).

A means of achieving positive health is through empowerment, the degree of which may be determined by an individual's level of control and participation. In addition the concept can be applied at community level directed at social and environmental change (Tones and Green, 2004; Mackereth, 2007; also see Case Study).

The Ottawa Charter defined the term 'health promotion' as 'the process of enabling people to increase control over the determinates of health and thereby improve their health' (WHO, 1986). It was the catalyst for increased momentum in distinguishing health promotion from public health as a discipline, and proposed three strategies for health promotion which have been successively built on:

- advocacy for health to create essential conditions for health;
- enabling all people to achieve their full health potential;
- mediating between different interests in society in pursuit of health.

Public health is defined as the science and art of promoting health, preventing disease, and prolonging life through the organised efforts of society (Acheson Report, 1998). The emphasis is on disease prevention, which covers measures to prevent disease occurring, such as risk factors, and also to arrest its progress and reduce its consequences once established (WHO, 1984).

Early examples of health education activities are strongly linked with public health efforts to combat squalor and provide clean water supplies in the earlier part of the twentieth century. There was an emphasis on giving personal information aimed at changing behaviour via educational and psychological means (Tones and Green, 2004). Debate continues about the merits and differences in approach between health promotion and health education which can be seen as both opposing and complementary. Whitehead (2003) suggests that nurses fail to conceptualise the differences and use the terms interchangeably, and need to be supported more specifically to practise within a health promotion framework. Both approaches address health but it is proposed that the setting, such as hospital, community or workplace, may influence the choice of approach used. Finally, health promotion includes efforts to tackle the social and environmental determinates of health by means of healthy public policy (Tones and Green, 2004).

Global and national policies should be considered for their potential impact on health and the development of local strategies. They will enable practitioners to justify and implement health promotion initiatives by embracing the most up to date approaches for groups and communities.

Box 27.1 Summary of UK Strategies and Policies influencing Health Promotion

- Health of the Nation (DH, 1992): CHD, cancer, mental illness, sexual health, accidents.

- The New NHS, Modern Dependable (DH, 1997): HIMPs, PCTs, HAZs.

- Saving Lives: Our Healthier Nation (DH, 1999): Focus on wider determinates of health.

- National Service Frameworks (DH, 1999 to date): CHD, MH, older people, diabetes, children.

- The NHS Plan (DH, 2000b): Developing primary care, screening, smoking cessation services, new initiatives: diet, cancer, heart disease, mental health, Sure Start.

- Choosing Health (DH, 2004b): Healthy choices, reduce inequalities.

(Continued)

- Our Health, Our Care, Our Say (DH, 2006e): New direction for community services.

- Essence of Care Benchmarks for Promoting Health (DH, 2006f): 9 benchmarks include empowerment, engagement and partnership.

- Our NHS, Our Future (DH, 2006e): Fair, personalised, effective and safe care.

Models of health promotion

Understanding different health promotion perspectives will help the practitioner choose an effective approach or strategy such as the bio-medical, behavioural or socio-environmental approach (Earle et al., 2007: 130). Various models of health promotion assist practitioners to integrate practice with theory, and to analyse and reflect on health promotion activities. Four examples are summarised in Table 27.1, each involving discrete stages or steps.

CASE STUDY

Community allotment schemes have been running across the UK for several years. Many were initiated through funding from health action zones.

Projects help people develop and share skills and learn about growing fruit and vegetables. Health benefits may be directly linked to consuming freshly grown produce. Increasing exercise as a result of sustained moderate digging has positive benefits on cardiovascular function. People can become involved for a few hours weekly or daily. Individuals may walk or cycle between home and allotment, instead of driving. For those with mobility restrictions, projects have provided wheelchair access, and paved and seating areas.

Opportunities to engage in social interactions develop people's confidence, increasing communication and social networking skills. Other advantages are the allotments' accessibility to all community members, from schoolchildren to the elderly, and those with mental health, physical or learning disabilities. This benefits all, as accessibility promotes social inclusion.

Table 27.1 *Models of health promotion*

Beattie's Model	4 strategies: Persuasion, personal counselling, legislative action and community development.
Tannahill's Model	The model combines prevention, health education and health protection.
Prochaska and Diclemente's Stages of Change (Transtheoretical) Model	Pre-contemplation, contemplation, readiness for action, action and maintenance.
Becker's Health Belief Model	Motivation to change depends on concern about perceived susceptibility and severity outweighed by belief in the benefits and effectiveness.

Source: adapted from Naidoo and Wills, 2000

The case study illustrates the benefits of health promotion activities that are facilitated through community action and empowerment. *Choosing Health* (DH, 2004b) promotes raising awareness and supporting the benefits of activity in early years, schools and communities, and encourages physical activities. There may, however, be psychological, behavioural and environmental barriers to overcome before taking up such activities.

CONCLUSION

The chapter has summarised the key theories, policies and debates concerning health promotion and its future direction.

From the public health perspective, the burden of disease is shifting from communicable to non-communicable diseases. Consequently health promotion is evolving as a defined specialism within public health, in order to address these changing needs through improving people's health and wellbeing.

FURTHER READING

Mackereth, C. (2007) *Community Development: New Challenges, New Opportunities.* London: CPHVA

WHO (1998b) *Health Promotion Glossary.* [Retrieved 2 April 2008, from http://www.who.int/hpr/NPH/docs/hp_glossary_en.pdf] Geneva: WHO.

public health and health promotion

28 Screening and Public Health

Mzwandile (Andi) Mabhala

DEFINITION

The original meaning of the word 'screen' was 'sieve', an apparatus used to separate bad corn from good (Simpson and Weiner, 1989). The 'sieve' concept is helpful because an inherent fact of screening is that the healthy population and the population with disease or its precursors are rarely completely discrete and separate populations like goats and sheep. Screening tests sort out the apparently well persons who probably have a disease from those who probably do not. Therefore, a commonly used definition of screening is the systematic application of a test or inquiry, to identify individuals at sufficient risk of a specific disorder to warrant further investigation or direct preventative action, amongst persons who have not sought medical attention on account of symptoms of that disorder (Miller and Vivek, 2004).

The UK National Screening Committee (2003) defines screening as a public health service in which members of a defined population – who do not necessarily perceive they are at risk of, or are already affected by, a disease or its complications – are asked questions or offered a test to identify those individuals who are more likely to be helped than harmed by further tests or treatment to reduce the risk of a disease or its complications.

These definitions emphasise two important ethical points: first, all screening examinations are preliminary and further investigation will be required to verify that those who screen positive really do have the abnormality and require treatment (true positives), and to eliminate those who screen positive but do not actually have the abnormality (false positives) (Holland et al., 2006); and secondly, those invited to participate in screening are not patients and most of them will not become patients.

- Information is a central concept in modern healthcare in general and screening in particular.
- Participation in screening is voluntary.
- Criteria must be applied before screening procedures are introduced.
- Ethical considerations, such as the harm-to-benefit ratio, are paramount.
- All screening examinations are preliminary.

DISCUSSION

General criteria for a screening programme

The guiding principles for instituting a screening programme were first produced by Wilson and Jungner (1968) and published as a World Health Organization monograph. After 39 years of existence this remains a landmark contribution to the screening literature (Holland et al., 2006). The principles are fundamental to the integrity of the screening process in any country, and (in their modified form) are considered below.

Appraisal and quality control

In any screening programme, as with any other service programme, adequate steps must be taken to ensure that the original objectives are being met and that the methodology meets appropriate standards. The ideal method for evaluating a screening programme is the randomised controlled trial (RCT) or systematic review of randomised controlled trials (Muir Gray, 2001; Holland et al., 2006). Difficult as they may be to organise, RCTs of public health interventions such as screening should be subjected to the same rigorous appraisal as is applied to clinical interventions. Indeed, it could be argued that there is a need for stronger evidence to support the introduction of screening as a public health intervention because it is offered to healthy populations. As no intervention is without risk, some of the people who are subject to it – a proportion of whom would not have developed the disease if the intervention had not been introduced – will be put at risk (Muir Gray, 2001).

Criteria for evaluation of screening

Evaluation must be an integral part of any screening procedure. A number of general criteria should be borne in mind when evaluating screening:

Table 28.1 *Criteria for a screening programme*

Disease	The disease prevalence should be high and the cause of substantial mortality and/or morbidity.
	The natural history of the condition should be known. Ideally, this implies that it is known at what stage in the disease process progression, disability and/or death can no longer be prevented.
	The disease should have a detectable preclinical phase.
	The disease should be treatable, and there should be a recognised treatment for abnormalities detected following screening.
	There should be evidence of effectiveness of treatment-detected abnormality.
The test	There should be a non-invasive test with high validity.
	A simple, cheap, safe, precise and reliable screening test should be used.
	The test should be acceptable to the population.
	There should be an agreed policy on the further diagnostic investigation of individuals with a positive test result and on the choices available to those individuals.
The diagnosis/treatment	The success of screening will depend upon the extent that those identified as having an abnormal test result accept the procedures offered to them for further evaluation, and the effectiveness of the therapy offered.

the test must be cheap, be simple to perform, easy to interpret and, where possible, capable of use by paramedics and other non-medical personnel. It should be *acceptable* to those undergoing it. It should be reliable; in other words, it should give consistent results in repeated trials. And most importantly it should be valid. By validity is meant the test's ability to measure or discover what the investigator wants it to (Beaglehole et al., 1993; Donaldson and Donaldson, 2003; Miller and Vivek, 2004). In other words, how good is the test in discriminating between people who have the disease and people who are healthy? Validity is usually expressed in terms of *sensitivity* and *specificity* (Beaglehole et al., 1993; Donaldson and Donaldson, 2003; Miller and Vivek, 2004).

To understand the validity of screening, it is helpful to look at it this way. Applying a screening test to a population may divide people into four possible types (Table 28.2): there may be (a) people who tested positive and have a disease (true positives), (b) people who tested

Table 28.2 *Sensitivity and specificity of a screening test*

	Disease present	Disease absent	Total
Positive test	a	b	a + b
Negative test	c	d	c + d
Total	a + c	b + d	a + b + c + d

positive but are free from the disease (false positives), (c) people who tested negative but have the disease (false negatives), and (d) people who tested negative and are free from the disease (true negatives). The concepts of sensitivity and specificity take account of these problems.

Sensitivity is the ability of a test to detect all those with the disease in the screened population. In other words, a very sensitive test would have no (or very few) missed cases (false negatives) (Donaldson and Donaldson, 2003).

Specificity is the ability of a test to identify correctly those who are free of the disease in the screened population. A highly specific test would have no (or few) people wrongly labelled as diseased (false positives). The ideal would be to have a screening test that was both 100 per cent sensitive and 100 per cent specific; however, a balance has to be struck between the two because the cut-off point between normal and abnormal is usually arbitrary.

CASE STUDY

Empathise with Mr and Mrs Ngubo. They spent months agonising about the arrival of their first-born. The arrival of a baby should be a moment of jubilation, but this wasn't so with the Ngubos. The agony began as they argued over the letter containing the triple test screening results.

'They say my baby's going to have Down's syndrome!' cried Mrs Ngubo.

'Who said that?' growled Mr Ngubo.

'It's the results from the blood test a student midwife took a few weeks ago,' replied his wife.

'Why did you consent to that nonsense? You should've asked what it was about before somebody poked you in the arm!' he yelled.

'She said there's a government directive that all pregnant women take this test,' his wife explained. 'They've invited us to see a consultant and offered another test called amnio which will confirm if my baby is

Down's, but there's a high risk of miscarriage.'

'What's the point of that?' Mr Ngubo demanded. 'What if the baby isn't Down's, but you miscarry it? What if the baby is Down's, then what are you going to do?'

'They offered us termination if the baby is confirmed to have Down's,' said his wife tearfully.

'Are you considering termination?' asked Mr Ngubo.

'Under no circumstances will I consider killing my baby,' snorted a defiant Mrs Ngubo.

Ethical considerations

The important ethical principles associated with screening pro-grammes are: doing more good than harm, informed consent and infor-mation. Although screening is often promoted as if it implies a benefit to everyone who is screened, in fact in some circumstances individuals included in screening programmes may be placed at a disadvantage – for example, individuals who have negative test results when they actually have the abnormality in question (false negatives). This obviously has serious implications, because individuals with negative test results will not normally be tested further. There may also be psychological con-sequences related to screening. The above scenario demonstrates an example of a couple who suffered psychological harm from being labelled as being at risk of having a Down's syndrome baby, when the treatment options were not acceptable to them because of their beliefs. This indicates that sometimes being labelled as being at risk of disease can be traumatic (Donaldson and Donaldson, 2003; Holland et al., 2006).

Another ethical dilemma for screening programmes is how to imple-ment informed consent. Information about the consequences of the test, the diagnostic assessment process, the disease to be detected and the treatments should be presented if a truly informed decision is to be made. Presenting such a large amount of information is obviously difficult in a busy healthcare setting. As appears to be the case in the scenario, the stu-dent failed to provide sufficient information to empower the participants to make an informed decision about the test and treatment options.

There is general consensus in the literature (Wilson and Jungner, 1968; Beaglehole et al., 1993; Muir Gray, 2001; Donaldson and Donaldson, 2003; UK National Screening Committee, 2003; Holland et al., 2006) that information is one of the central concepts in modern healthcare in general and screening in particular. In practice, however, there are some instances when information involves nothing more than providing a leaflet and possibly offering a brief discussion with a health professional, with the emphasis on achieving a positive response (Miller and Vivek, 2004). This is not enough. Sometimes the participants may require special education (as shown in the scenario) so that they understand the whole diagnostic process, in order to reduce anxiety accompanying the identification of an abnormality and to ensure that they comply with the recommendations for management.

CONCLUSION

It is increasingly recognised from a growing evidence base that, when applied systematically, screening has real potential to improve the public's health. However, the technical ability to perform a screening procedure does not guarantee its ethical acceptability. More than ever before, it is vital that the implementation of screening programmes is based on strong scientific evidence, and that rigorous criteria are applied and ethical principles adhered to.

FURTHER READING

Miller, A.B. and Vivek, G. (2004) *Screening*, 4th edn. Oxford: Oxford University Press.
UK National Screening Committee (2003) *Criteria for appraising the viability effectiveness and appropriateness of a screening programme*. Retrieved 12, December 2007, from http://www.library.nhs.uk/screening/

screening and public health

29 Disease Prevention

Alan Massey

DEFINITION

Disease prevention is a central pillar of public health practice. Classically, disease prevention is a biomedical approach aimed at addressing the burden of ill health. Within the biomedical framework disease prevention has three phases: primary, secondary and tertiary.

Prevention may be accomplished in the pre-disease state by measures designed to promote general optimum health or by the specific protection of human beings against disease agents or the establishment of barriers against agents in the environment. These procedures have been termed primary prevention. As soon as the disease is detectable, early in pathogenesis, secondary prevention may be accomplished by early diagnosis and prompt and adequate treatment. When the process of pathogenesis has progressed and the disease has advanced beyond its early stages, secondary prevention may also be accomplished by means of adequate treatment to prevent and limit disability. Later, when defect and disability have been fixed, tertiary prevention may be accomplished by rehabilitation (Leavell and Clarke, 1965: 20).

KEY POINTS

- Influence of the biomedical model on disease prevention.
- Primary, secondary and tertiary approaches to disease prevention.
- Application of the epidemiological triangle in the management of disease processes and prevention.
- Role of health promotion, education and individual health behaviours.
- Influence of policy drivers on disease prevention strategies.

DISCUSSION

Prevention, although utilised since early antiquity, significantly developed during the epidemiological revolution of the nineteenth century. At this time reduction in morbidity and mortality was achieved through social and environmental reforms in hygiene, housing, sanitation and working conditions (Rogers, 2003). Changes in morbidity and mortality shifted the focus of health policies away from disease to health behaviours and led to the rise in health education. This aimed to inform individuals about the outcomes of risky health behaviours. In the latter part of the twentieth century a reawakening of the effectiveness of disease prevention occurred within public health. The rationale for this development lies in an understanding of the 'prevention paradox'. According to Baggott (2000) preventative measures which benefit the population have little appeal to each individual. This means that left to their own devices, individuals have little incentive to contribute to activities that improve their health. Therefore, measures aimed at the individual should be replaced or enhanced by greater influence from the state to address the public's health. To support this paradox is a greater understanding that the preventative model, which focuses on individualism and which takes little account of the determinants of health, can cause an increase in health inequalities. Those in privileged positions will attain better health than those dependent on the state for health interventions (Tones and Green, 2004).

Individualism has been superseded by socialist ideologies as the dominant approach to addressing ill health. This ideological shift means that greater emphasis is now placed on disease prevention through legislative action and via the reorganisation of health services to address health issues. Depending on one's ideological viewpoint prevention can be viewed as an egalitarian act or as an oppressive mechanism of social control.

The basic premise for undertaking disease prevention can be understood by an awareness of the epidemiological triangle (see Figure 29.1).

An agent may be thought of as a substance that must be present for a disease or condition to occur. Transmission of an agent to a host may be accomplished in a variety of ways: infectious agents such as bacteria, viruses and parasites by contact; chemical agents such as toxic chemicals or pesticides may be inhaled, or absorbed through the skin; poisons may be ingested.

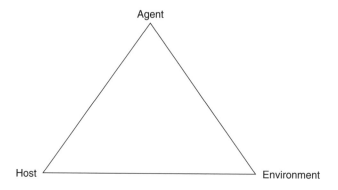

Figure 29.1 *Disease triad*

Environmental factors include climate (temperature, rainfall); plant and animal life (agents, reservoirs or habitats for agents); human population distribution (crowding, social support, resources, and access to care); and working conditions (stress, noise, job satisfaction).

Host factors concern the health status of the human and include genetic susceptibility; immutable and age/gender, characteristics; immunology status; lifestyle factors; diet and exercise.

Prevention strategies are ones which seek to address these factors either individually or concurrently. Changes in one of the elements of the triangle can influence the occurrence of disease by increasing or decreasing a person's risk. Risk is understood as the probability an individual will become ill. Reducing or eliminating this probability is the goal of prevention. The power of the biomedical approach to disease prevention can be seen by examining the reduction in communicable disease; for example, smallpox was responsible for an estimated 300–500 million deaths in the twentieth century. Following improvement of the host's immune system via vaccination, smallpox was eradicated in 1979 (WHO, 2000).

In critiquing disease prevention model, Baggott (2000) informs us that the biomedical approach generalises health behaviours to a focus on danger and risk. This leads to a requirement for greater surveillance and attempts to orientate health behaviours to health outcomes. This process however adopts a victim-blaming approach, where the individual concerned is blamed for health outcomes, due to their own risky behaviour. No consideration is given to the social, environmental and political factors that influence health choices.

Despite its lack of universal acceptance the re-emergence of disease prevention was enacted via *Prevention and Health: Everybody's Business* (DHSS, 1976). This set out areas for disease prevention and linked health promotion to addressing health behaviours. Within this format health problems are an outcome of lifestyles and the risks we choose. This approach dominated partly because of the realisation that the problems facing society at that time were the diseases of affluence; i.e. the factors which cause disease are ones we ourselves choose: for example, lack of exercise or poor diet, smoking. The process of addressing risk attracts criticism as society's attitude to biomedical science and risk is declining. The limitations of the biomedical model are explored by Tones and Green (2004), who inform us that the biomedical model is based in the technical rational school of thought which reduces health to a mechanistic process where specific diseases have specific causes. The difficulty with this ideology is that it does not pay enough attention to the other sociological factors which determine our health. There is at the present time a lack of consensus on which determinants of health need addressing. Reaching a consensus is a difficult undertaking in modern society, according to Orme et al. (2007). Authoritarian policy creation, target setting and implementation are increasingly seen as paternalistic and lacking in relevance to societies' needs. Society in general is more sophisticated in its understanding that science can be utilised to over-emphasise risk and to manipulate behaviour. The declining consensus among biomedical experts translates into a lack of congruence of risks outlined with the lived experiences of individuals (Baggott, 2000). To address these processes biomedical approaches to prevention should be supported by sociological actions to address determinants of disease in a manner which reflects societal needs. In addition, the biomedical model focuses on a negative view of health in which absence of disease is the priority. It is limited in its understanding of factors which affect the quality of life (Davies and Macdowall, 2006). In an effort to avoid this emphasis, primary prevention can be utilised to shift the focus to prevention rather than cure.

Focusing on risk however is not without merit. It is a useful mechanism for strategic planners as it allows them to target health interventions (Davies and Macdowall, 2006). Focusing on risks leads to addressing health issues via monitoring, controlling, prioritising and targeting actions to reduce risk (Tones and Green, 2004). Targeting is a useful tool, according to Davies and Macdowall (2006), as the setting of health targets is a key mechanism in raising the aspirations of society and for delivering improvements.

CASE STUDY

Diane is a middle-aged IT manager; she is middle class and her risk of contracting a non-communicable disease is seen as minimal. The biggest threats to her health are those she chooses to undertake. She eats a healthy diet and exercises regularly. She does not smoke; however, due to the pressures of work she drinks one bottle of wine per day. She also utilises illegal drugs on an infrequent basis to help her in times of difficulty. To address her problems broad public health policy should be adopted together with targeted health counselling to deal with risk factors in an integrated way, tackling both behavioural and environmental risks. This broad brush approach should include measures such as disease prevention and health promotion; incentives for prevention; screening; rapid intervention; educational programmes; control of environmental and occupational stressors and organisation of health services to address health in a proactive fashion.

CONCLUSION

In response the World Health Organization (WHO) took the lead in providing a united approach to prevention within the Health for All, 2000 programme. The WHO sets out targets for prevention in its consecutive document *Health for All by 2021* (WHO, 1985). The rationale for this approach is that while preventative interventions have resulted in overall health improvements, preventable illness and injury continue to place a burden of disease on society in respect of health, quality of living and cost-effectiveness.

This burden is clarified by the Centers for Disease Control in America (CCDC, 2007) which informs us that preventable illness accounts for up to 90 per cent of morbidity statistics and for eight of the ten leading causes of mortality. The picture is similar in the United Kingdom and the burden of disease is predominated by respiratory disease, cancers, circulatory diseases, communicable and non-communicable diseases, accidents and mental health problems (http://www.statistics.gov.uk, accessed November 2007). The vast majority of disease in this country is now non-communicable in nature and too many people are dying prematurely or are being made ill when the means of preventing this is known.

FURTHER READING

Baggott, R. (2000) *Public Health: Policy and Politics*. Basingstoke: Palgrave Macmillan.

Davies, M. and Macdowall, W. (2006) *Health Promotion Theory*. Maidenhead: Open University Press.

Tones, K. and Green, J. (2004) *Health Promotion: Planning Strategies*. London: Sage.

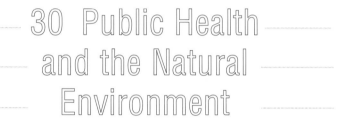

30 Public Health and the Natural Environment

Kim Greening

Both nature and the natural environment have central importance to the lives of people; to their health, to their wellbeing and to the role played in the sustainable development of their habitat.

DEFINITION

In the Australian State of the Environment Report (2001) the natural environment is defined as 'an environment that is not the result of human activity or intervention'. This definition is both helpful and problematic because what we take to be natural has often been shaped by humans; large areas of Britain would in their natural state be forested and as Schama (1995) writes of Yosemite, 'the brilliant meadow-floor which suggested to its first eulogists a pristine Eden was in fact the result of regular fire-clearances by its Ahwahneechee Indian occupants'.

A difference is often established between the natural environment and the built environment. However, focusing on the boundaries between the natural and the built environment in order to develop understanding is also problematic (the latter relates to buildings and structures that have been designed and constructed by humans). For example green spaces such as formal parks and gardens within cities can be viewed as being manufactured structures, i.e. the built environment, whereas city railway embankments are viewed otherwise because they are naturally colonised by flora and fauna.

KEY POINTS

- There is an innate link between good public health and natural environment.
- Natural environment plays a key role in healthy emotional and physical development in childhood.
- Early childhood exposure to natural environment improves their awareness of risks associated with nature.

DISCUSSION

In 1964 Erich Fromm proposed the term 'biophilia' to describe a *psychological orientation* of being attracted to all that is alive and vital. Twenty years later this term was popularised by Edward Wilson, a naturalist based at Harvard University. Wilson believed that knowing living things well elevated the very concept of life (Wilson, 1984).

It is in early childhood that many people first develop a love of nature. Maria Montessori (1976) wrote of the importance of using nature as a source of inspiration for learning. The outdoors was recognised as an enriching environment for child development and Montessori recommended that children were taken into nature for first-hand experiences.

Forty years ago, in the 1960s, children spent a higher proportion of time outdoors. The local copse, woodland stream or nearby park were all areas children explored. Ball games and other activities such as skipping and 'British Bulldog' took place on spare ground or in the street. The child's play horizons were not confined to the immediate area near the home. A decline in outdoor physical play and the corresponding decrease in mobility amongst children has been explored by Wheway and Millward (1997) who note a measurable detrimental effect on children's physical health.

Today children spend more time indoors watching television and sitting in front of computer screens or PlayStations. The increased technology in the lives of children appears to be associated with the rise in obesity. The National Childhood Obesity Database 2005–2006 (DH, 2007c) reveals that for reception class children (4–5-year-olds) 21.5 per cent of girls and 24.1 per cent of boys are now classed as either overweight or obese. The results of a randomised control trial, undertaken by Robinson (2001), concluded that 'television viewing is a cause of increased body fatness and that reducing television viewing is a promising strategy for preventing childhood obesity'.

In his book *Last Child in the Woods: Saving Our Children from Nature-Deficit Disorder* Richard Louv (2005) reveals the growing body of evidence which shows that direct contact with nature is essential for healthy physical and emotional development in childhood. Louv advocates that parents should try to reconnect their children with nature as the benefits include psychological wellbeing, self-confidence and better body image.

Many parents are, however, over-protective and worry about the perceived dangers in the outdoor environment; they are becoming overly risk-averse. As Tim Gill (2005), a leading adviser on childhood, comments:

Fear of traffic risks and 'stranger danger' are holding our children captive indoors. For the sake of their health and development and for the environment they will one day need to protect we have to find ways of getting them into the wild.

To learn about the risks associated with the natural world children need to experience it. For example if they walk across seaweed strewn rocks at the beach they will learn about the slippery properties of wet seaweed. Similarly, baking jacket potatoes on an open fire teaches a child about the dangers of hot embers. Learning about hazards in an acceptable and controlled way is the approach advocated by the Royal Society for the Prevention of Accidents. The Society strongly supports the idea that engaging with risk is an essential part of safety education for every child (Bibbings, 2007).

Our early childhood experiences shape and define our adult life. There is evidence to show that emotional affinity with nature can be traced to present and past experiences in natural environments (Kals and Montada, 1999). This is an important finding given the environmental issues that individuals and societies will have to face in the mid-twenty-first century.

Inactivity amongst the adult population is a major public health problem. People who are physically inactive increase their risk of coronary heart disease, stroke and type 2 diabetes and thereby run a greater risk of premature death. The Department of Health (2004b) recommends 30 minutes of moderate activity at least five days a week. In a report undertaken for the Royal Society for the Protection of Birds, William Bird (2004) a former general practitioner examines whether green space and biodiversity can increase levels of physical activity. His analysis of the evidence reveals important conclusions, including the following:

- Green space in an urban environment can improve life expectancy and decrease health complaints.
- For most people attendance at a gym does not provide the best way of increasing and sustaining physical activity.
- Physical activity specialists in the National Health Service need to be aware of the potential of green space.
- Good design of wildlife-rich gardens can be used to increase physical activity in sedentary and vulnerable patients or residents.
- The motivation to continue physical activity schemes is more likely to be sustained through the natural environment.
- There is a need for imaginative ways to promote a wildlife-rich green space, and for it to be marketed to different age groups.

To address the poor physical health of some of his overweight patients William Bird developed and promoted the idea of the Green Gym. Green Gyms are 'schemes that support people in gardening or local environmental improvement while providing opportunities for exercise and developing social networks' (DH, 2004a). The concept of the Green Gym is important because the activities involved have purpose, i.e. exercise is secondary to environmental and social benefits and it appears that this is more sustainable (Bird, 2004).

The value of the natural environment for psychological and mental wellbeing has recently received renewed recognition in the field of mental health. In the report *Ecotherapy: The Green Agenda for Mental Health* (Mind, 2007) the benefits of green exercise in the form of gardening, walking, conservation work, running and cycling have been explored.

Green exercise programmes are seen as treatment options for those with mental distress, i.e. clinically valid options that can play a vital part in patients' recovery (Mind, 2007). The report includes in its list of recommendations a call for access to green space to be a part of care planning and assessment and for GPs to consider referring patients for green exercise.

CASE STUDY

Founded in the United States in 1996, Casting for Recovery came to the United Kingdom and Ireland in 2006. Casting for Recovery is a non-profit support and educational programme for women who have or have had breast cancer. Weekend retreats incorporate counselling, educational services and the sport of fly fishing to promote mental and physical healing. The retreats provide an avenue for social support and group interactions, reducing the feeling of isolation many survivors might have. The dynamics of fly fishing provide a healing connection to the natural world, relieving everyday stress and promoting a sense of calm. Fly fishing techniques provide a gentle exercise for joint and soft tissue mobility. The retreats offer a forum for women with similar experiences to meet, learn a new skill and gain a respite from their everyday concerns. Further information can be obtained at www.castingforrecovery.org.uk

CONCLUSION

Obesity, inactivity and mental health problems are some of the major public health challenges to address in the twenty-first century. There is an emerging body of evidence to show that connectivity with nature and the natural environment has a positive influence on health and wellbeing and has a place in the practice of health professionals.

FURTHER READING

Bird, W. (2004) *Natural fit. Can green space and biodiversity increase levels of physical activity?* (Royal Society for the Protection of Birds). Retrieved 10 December 2007, from http://www.rspb.org/Images/natural_fit_full_version_tcm9-133055.pdf

Casting for Recovery (2008) Casting for recovery. Retrieved 20 March 2008, from www.castingforrecovery.org.uk

Natural England (2008) Natural England works for people, places and nature to conserve and enhance biodiversity, landscapes and wildlife in rural, urban, coastal and marine areas. Retrieved 3 April 2008, from http://www.naturalengland.org.uk

31 Environment and Public Health

Alex G. Stewart and Richard Jarvis

DEFINITION

There are three standard uses of the term 'environment':

1 *the natural environment*: air, water and land, with consideration to its biological, chemical and radiological composition and properties;
2 *the built environment*: residences, industrial and commercial sites and mobile sites, including road and air traffic, rail and sea movement;
3 *the social environment*: moving from the individual in ever increasing circles through family, friends and the workplace to the wider society and culture, with international influences having possible effects on all levels.

These meanings have arisen and are widely used in sustainable development and the prevention and mitigation of effects of climate change. Here, people and communities are viewed as being integral to the wider environment and their health as integral to the health of the environment. Public health actions, particularly in health protection and social equity, thus have the dual benefit of improving the health of communities and the health of the environment (Figure 31.1).

Unfortunately, many practitioners consider only the first, standard usage. But human public health and the health of the environment cannot be viewed or managed in isolation.

KEY POINTS

- Perceptions of risk and the risk of disease are different.
- Anxiety may be the biggest problem caused by most environmental hazards in the developed world.
- A strong multi-agency group will lead to a robust response.
- Good and clear communication with partners and public is vital.

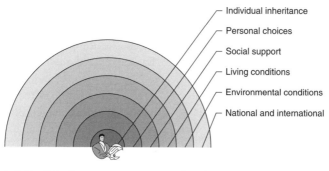

Individual inheritance	-	sex, age, genetic makeup
Personal choices	-	diet, smoking, alcohol and illicit drugs, other lifestyle choices
Social support	-	family, friends, colleagues, local community
Living conditions	-	home, water supply, sewerage, employment, health care, peace/war
Environmental conditions	-	working environment, quality of food source and supply, schooling
National and international	-	economy, religion and culture, trade, transport, natural world

Figure 31.1 *Determinants of health*

(Adapted from Stewart et al., 2005)

DISCUSSION

Consideration of the environment as a danger to health starts with identifying a hazard and assessing the risk to health from it. A hazard is a potential threat to health, while a risk is a quantified estimation of that threat. Large hazards might pose small risks, such as toxic chemicals stored on a well regulated and well run industrial site, while small hazards, such as the exhaust emissions from a single car, might pose a large risk when found in quantity in a town centre.

The environment can be supportive of, or improve, human health, rather than simply detracting from it. Furthermore, a particular setting in the environment can be both a hazard to health and act to improve health at the same time (see Case Studies).

Land, air and water can all be contaminated with chemicals. The evidence for risk of disease from residence near landfill sites is subject to debate (Vrijheid, 2000; Food Standards Agency, 2002). There is no convincing evidence that contaminated land in the UK has caused ill health, although in other parts of the world contaminated land has had a serious impact (Kibble and Saunders, 2001).

The evidence for air pollution affecting health is stronger. Clear associations have been reported between both daily and long-term average concentrations of air pollutants and effects on the cardiovascular system (COMEAP, 2006).

Overall, anxiety is probably the biggest health problem from the environment in developed countries. For example, the two largest radiation risks in the UK are cancer caused by exposure to radon gas and sunlight (UV). However, public concern about radiation is focused on mobile phones and phone masts, which probably pose a very low risk, if any. Smells and noise are often causes of anxiety rather than disease.

Analysis

For a better understanding of hazards and risks, a source–pathway–receptor link is needed. If one or more of these three is missing then there can be no threat to health. To public health practitioners, the only receptor is the population, while environmental scientists consider non-human receptors. Pathways identify the way the pollutant moves to the receptor from a variety of sources, e.g. through the air or the diet from industrial sites, traffic pollution or fires.

As well as looking at hazards and risk, public health practitioners need also to look at diseases and syndromes that might have environmental causes or which are modified, either positively or negatively, by an environmental factor.

In practice, the majority of incidents are situations where either:

- A hazard (source) is present and some contingency creates a pathway and leads to potential exposure of receptors. Typical examples of this include acute exposure following a spill at a factory, or chronic exposure to emissions from a landfill. The purpose of investigating is to establish the degree of hazard by understanding the specific toxicology and epidemiology
- An excess of a given disease or syndrome is noted, an environmental cause is suspected, and a source–pathway–receptor linkage may exist. Such 'clusters' may be real or perceived and the aim of the investigation is to (1) establish the degree of excess of illness (if any) and (2) assess the likelihood of an environmental exposure being responsible, compared to the likelihood of other possible explanations. The investigation is best approached in a step-wise fashion (King et al., 1993), to ensure that resources are used wisely.

In both types of incident, the investigation will point to means to prevent or reduce further exposure and to manage the ongoing health needs of those affected. As with any public health action, it is important that investigation and control are undertaken in conjunction with other stakeholders, usually the emergency services, the health service and local authorities.

The information on which to base a response is often limited. Good toxicological information is limited to 5,000 chemicals out of 31 million known. Likewise, epidemiological studies can be difficult to undertake, due to effects such as small numbers, mobility of population, difficulties in case definition or clustering problems. Incidence, prevalence, cohort and case-control studies can be useful if their limitations are appreciated (Gordis, 2005).

Response

The response to any environmental situation should

1   gather and confirm information on sources, pathways and receptors;
2   control, with others, the appropriate aspects to contain the situation;
3   communicate and collaborate with stakeholders and others.

Some of these might happen simultaneously. A framework (Figure 31.2) for achieving this will place variable emphasis on the three strands, depending on the incident being managed. However, all strands need to be considered to produce a robust, multi-agency response, especially since decisions about the response are often based on sub-optimal information.

The key skill in response is public health; the scale of the response will vary (see Box 31.1).

Box 31.1   Increasing levels of response to environmental situations

1   *Level One*: Telephone advice or information given or put in post/email.

2   *Level Two*: Report written and sent to enquirer.

3   *Level Three*: Short meeting held with other agencies to agree a joint plan of action.

4   *Level Four*: More formal, Health Protection Advisory Group meets, often several times, to plan and run a multi-dimensional investigation and response.

(Adapted from Reid et al., 2005)

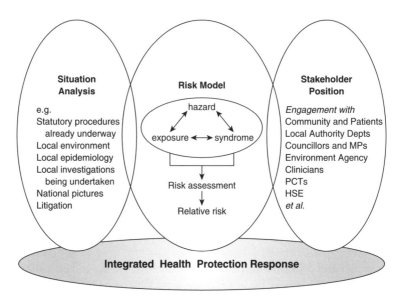

Figure 31.2 *The components of a good response to an environmental situation (Adapted from Reid et al., 2005)*

CASE STUDIES

Health risk v. health gain

Following investigation into contamination in a stream running through a golf course, the golf-course topsoil was found to contain hazardous concentrations of arsenic. A multi-agency group decided to close the course, pending remediation. However, the golf course remained closed for a number of years, with the resulting loss of amenities and health gain to golfers and others who used the course for walking.

The balancing of different health needs and risks can be very difficult in practice.

As a result of the lessons learned from the golf course, when the sports field of a primary school was found to be built on contaminated land, it was possible to resist calls for closure of the site. Use of the sports field was controlled to reduce children's exposure to the soil and remediation was deemed unnecessary.

A behavioural approach was found to be the best means to control a chemical hazard.

Risk perception and communication

A major fire in a brewery resulted in a plume of asbestos downwind of the brewery across a residential area. Residents were concerned about health effects from exposure to any deposit of asbestos or from airborne dust.

Asbestos fibres become denatured when exposed to temperatures above 450°C in a fire, turning from a high hazard to a low hazard. Lumps of asbestos are not a hazard since they do not release fibres.

Residents were advised about the presence of asbestos. They were encouraged to avoid raising dust, and told to lift large pieces using plastic bags and put them in their household waste. Specialists were called to clean the streets and gardens of obvious contamination. Some residents remained concerned despite these reassurances.

Communicating the risk, or lack of it, to a community in an acute situation is not easy, requiring good public health judgement (Bennett and Calman, 1999).

A perceived cluster

Residents opposed to the positioning of a mobile phone mast claimed a large number of cases of cancer in its vicinity. On investigation there was found to be no excess of any particular type of cancer. In fact, the total number of all cancers was not raised.

Had there been an excess of a particular cancer, knowledge about aetiology of cancer would suggest that exposure to mobile phone radiation is far less likely as a cause than lifestyle factors, e.g. smoking, diet or exercise.

CONCLUSION

Public health can lead investigation into and response to environmental problems in a robust and satisfactory manner. The local community can be given reassurance that their environment is not only safe to live in but enhances their quality of life.

FURTHER READING

Health Protection Agency (2007) *Chemical hazards and poisons division*. Retrieved 31 July 2007, from http://www.hpa.org.uk/chemicals/default.htm

Health Protection Agency (2007) *Radiation protection division*. (On ionising and non-ionising radiation). Retrieved 31 July 2007, from http://www.hpa.org.uk/radiation/default.htm

environment and public health

32 Emergency and Disaster Planning

Walid El Ansari and Pat Deeny

DEFINITION

Disaster is a calamitous event of slow or rapid onset that results in large-scale physical destruction of property, social infrastructure and human life. It overwhelms the existing resources and coping mechanisms of individuals, groups, communities and societies. A disaster's impact is determined by the nature of the physical event, loss of life, level of disease and destruction of property. The lack of preparedness and poor infrastructure make an equal contribution to the overall impact of the disaster (Deeny et al., 2007). Quarantelli (1998) outlines the importance of the imbalance in the 'demand–capability ratio'. This 'imbalance' between the ability of the individual, group or community to cope with the event is central to understanding the concept of 'disaster'.

KEY POINTS

- Natural and human-initiated disasters remain the greatest threat to human life. While it is difficult to predict exactly when a disaster might occur, assessment of the vulnerability of communities to disasters is important.
- Many disasters occur in developing countries with poor public health infrastructure.
- Due to political and ethnic conflicts such disasters often develop into complex emergencies.
- Disasters comprise distinct phases each impacting on the social, economic and cultural activities causing increased community dysfunction, disruptions of social fabric and mental morbidity.
- Dealing with the immediate and longer-term effects of disasters requires multi-agency partnerships.

174

DISCUSSION

Disasters: types and burdens

Most disasters are natural events (floods, earthquakes, hurricanes). However, other disasters are 'human-initiated', man-made or brought about by human activity (e.g. air crashes, war, bombings, mass murder, ethnic cleansing and even famine). Increasingly, disasters are attributed to human activity especially if we consider disasters as a result of global warming, use of nuclear weapons or chemicals, or creation of synthetic viruses. Whilst a famine is normally due to crop failure, the contributory factors are human-initiated such as failure of a country to provide proper resources, to prevent famine, or as in southern Sudan, an attempt by one ethnic group to force another on to land that cannot support adequate crops.

Acute disasters are the most widely reported (floods, bombings, terrorist attacks, wars, pandemics). 'Big events' that result in massive loss of life make headline news. Slower disasters receive less coverage but are equally devastating (famine, AIDS epidemics, malaria epidemics, or the increase in lifestyle diseases).

During the last decade of the twentieth century, about 75,250 people per annum across the world died as a result of natural or human-initiated disasters. During the same period, 210 million people per annum were affected by disasters (IFRC, 2001). Ryan et al. (2002) list 38 natural disasters of the twentieth century to emphasise the scale of human loss. Approximately 18 million lives were lost in these events (not including any wars that occurred).

About 300,000 people worldwide died as result of disasters in 2004 (IFRC, 2005). Statistics are influenced by the Indian Ocean tsunami (26 December 2004) when over 280,000 people died/went missing and 2 million people were affected. 'Global warming' and its impact on vulnerable communities/regions with endemic health problems (Oxfam, 2007), global terrorism, nuclear armaments and pandemics (Deeny et al., 2007) suggest that natural or human-initiated disasters remain the foremost threat to humans.

Coping with disasters: resilience and vulnerability

Resilience is the ability of individuals/communities to respond and adapt in a positive manner to negative life experiences. Hence, in a disaster, healthcare professionals need to identify the prerequisites to resilience, and be able to draw upon existing coping resources, knowledge and skills which exist within communities. These range from knowledge of the area and culture(s), to the communities' experience of previous disasters (Deeny and McFetridge, 2005). The identified coping resources can be enhanced, thereby empowering the community to cope with the disaster's impact.

Vulnerability describes the factors that impair individual/community responses in a disaster. Public health professionals need to consider vulnerabilities alongside resilience. Vulnerability may be the underpinning justification for intervention, and from a preparedness perspective, it is important to know the community's vulnerabilities. Vulnerabilities range from the 'risk of a disaster occurring' in the first place to the 'inability of the community to respond appropriately'. Disasters in the developing world illustrate the 'resilience–vulnerability' continuum (Deeny and McFetridge, 2005). Some communities, like individuals, are better at coping than others.

Phases of disasters

Pre-disaster period This refers to the weeks/days before a disaster occurs. It involves putting actions in place to mitigate loss of life, spread of disease, property damage and communications breakdown. In some disasters (hurricanes, floods) where it is known that the disaster will occur, this period is critical as communities can be evacuated and/or prepared by stocking up food and water, creating temporary shelters and toilet facilities and protecting vulnerable community members.

Acute or emergency phase This refers to the actual event (bomb, flood, explosion, earthquake) with mass casualties, injuries and loss of life and demand on emergency services. Casualties may be trapped and chaos/mayhem ensue. Local people at the scene immediately attempt to rescue survivors. If displacement of people from the area has not occurred in the pre-disaster period it will occur at this stage. Hurried movement at/from the disaster scene leads to children getting separated from parents, and to road traffic accidents. This phase is normally over in 12 hours but it may last for days if the threat of further events is still present. Earthquakes may go on for days where aftershocks are as devastating as the first 'quake'.

Post-acute phase This is the time after the main event. Although the threat of the disaster has subsided, not all survivors may have been accounted for and communications (roads, rail, telephones, electricity) may not have been re-established. As most disasters, especially man-made disasters (bombings, etc.) are treated as a 'crime scene', the police and other investigators will be gathering evidence. From a public health perspective, this phase presents problems associated with disease, as disasters disrupt water/sewerage systems (typhoid, cholera), and large numbers of displaced people gather (respiratory illness, influenza, measles).

During this phase the dead are buried. Psychosocial interventions (e.g. counselling) are not really necessary, as communities are normally cohesive, helpful and supportive. 'Watchful waiting' means that healthcare professionals do not interfere immediately.

Recovery phase This is after the post-acute phase when the community is trying to get back to normal. It includes reflections on what happened and dealing with the loss. Counselling/psychosocial support is always required; families and community groups are helped to come to terms with the loss and talk through their experiences. Post traumatic stress disorder can develop in some individuals. This phase may last for years if the threat of further disasters is still present or there is no resource to help communities 'get back on their feet'. The anniversaries of the event can be traumatic and individuals/families require additional support. Mourning can last for many years.

Post-recovery phase This is when the community is 'back to normal'. However, there is debate as to whether or not a community ever recovers from a disaster. The community now needs to begin planning for prevention of further disasters.

The final phase of the disaster is really the pre-disaster phase where the focus is again on disaster prevention/mitigation. Therefore the concept of disaster is cyclical (Figure 32.1).

CASE STUDY

Double Jeopardy: Disasters on Top of Poverty

The developing world (where the 'majority' of people live) is vulnerable to disasters and has little resources to cope with the effects. This

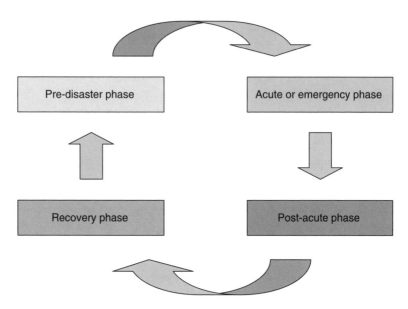

Figure 32.1 *Disasters as a cyclical process*

is complicated by globalisation whereby wealthier countries exploit developing technology to become wealthier and the poorer countries struggle in their wake (Deeny et al., 2007),

Of the 2,557 natural disasters in 1990–2000, 50 per cent were in countries of medium human development. Two thirds of those killed were from low human development countries and less than 30 per cent from medium human development countries (only 2 per cent were from highly developed countries). On average, 22.5 people die per disaster in highly developed nations, 145 people in medium development nations, while each disaster in low human development countries claims about 1,052 people (IFRC, 2001).

Poorer countries may experience a 'slow' disaster over months/years, but as devastating as a sudden disaster. The Burma cyclone is a typical example of double jeopardy whereby the poorest population group carry unfair burden of disaster. Burma is one of the poorest nations in south-eastern Asia, suffering from decades of stagnation, mismanagement and isolation. Coping with May 2008 tropical cyclone was compounded by poor public health infrastructure and poor government relation with the international community.

CONCLUSION

Disasters mean that a community may not be able to provide the individual with the resources to deal with such extraordinary events. Life after a disaster is different from before, requiring communities to adapt. The psychosocial processes experienced by those impacted by a disaster are similar to the normal coping mechanisms that are employed by humans in the face of any adversity. However, the scale of loss can be greater and extraordinary coping mechanisms may be required. Survival of a disaster affects the psychological, social, cultural and spiritual totality of the human being for weeks to years after the event. Disasters cause social and family disruptions, thereby causing further distress.

Vulnerable groups (older people, children, women, the disabled or mentally ill) are at risk. Healthcare workers must be aware of such groups within the community and must target and advocate for such groups during a disaster. Dealing with the immediate and the longer-term effects of disasters requires twofold action. First, that public health and other professionals are aware of the concepts associated with disaster response and preparedness in order to competently provide care and support. Such preparedness requires skills, training and development. Secondly, no single agency is able to deal with a disaster in isolation. Responses to disasters are inter-agency multi-sectoral activities. Public health professionals must collaborate with other involved organisations (voluntary and professional) in a co-ordinated overall response that takes the form of multi-agency partnerships at local, national and international levels.

FURTHER READING

Moore, T. and Lakha, R. (2006) *Tolley's Handbook of Disaster and Emergency Management: Principles and Practice*, 3rd edn. Oxford: Butterworth-Heinemann.

emergency and disaster planning

Edward Andersson and Walid El Ansari

DEFINITION

Despite its importance in healthcare there is no established shared definition of user involvement. User involvement can be interpreted as a wide range of activities, from the involvement of patients in individual treatment decisions and regimes, through patient consultation to the lobbying of collective organisations to influence health policy decisions (Andersson et al., 2006). Public involvement is the involvement of people in their wider role as citizens in healthcare decision-making. User involvement is the involvement of people in their role as current or future patients. In theory the former is motivated by the greater good as represented by health commissioning decisions, whereas the latter is taken to be motivated more by self-interest, aimed at improving services and treatment outcomes (Weale, 2006).

KEY POINTS

- User involvement is an important concept in healthcare.
- Successful involvement requires clear objectives which are communicated clearly to all parties.
- Increased user involvement challenges the traditional role of healthcare professionals.
- The effects of involvement are hard to measure. It can lead to a number of benefits for users.

DISCUSSION

User involvement has been discussed at least since the 1970s but only became an important concept in health policy in the mid-1990s. The term means different things to different people. Involvement takes place

INFORM	CONSULT	INVOLVE	COLLABORATE	EMPOWER
Public participation goal:	Public participation goal:	Public participation goal:	Public participation goal:	Public participation goal:
To provide the public with balanced and objective information to assist them in understanding the problem, alternatives, opportunities and/or solutions	To obtain public feedback on analysis, alternatives and/or decisions	To work directly with the public throughout the process to ensure that public concerns and aspirations are consistently understood and considered	To partner with the public in each aspect of the decision including the development of alternatives and the identification of the preferred solution	To place final decision-making in the hands of the public

Figure 33.1 *Levels of involvement (Source: Involve, 2005)*

on a continuum from information provision to empowerment, and from consultation to co-production, delegated power, and ultimate control of decisions (Involve, 2005; see Figure 33.1). User involvement describes many activities, ranging from the involvement of patients in treatment decisions, through patient consultation and lay members serving on advocacy committees, to the collective actions of organisations to influence policy-makers.

Involvement is undertaken for varied reasons. Distinctions are made between 'management-centred' involvement where managers define the agenda and 'user-centred' involvement; between involvement as a right; involvement as an instrumental way of achieving efficiency and improved health outcomes in healthcare; and between individual (choice) and collective (voice) user involvement (Harrison and Mort, 1998).

User involvement is in the UK often included in 'Patient and Public Involvement' (PPI). Public involvement relates to accountability for the spending of tax money and ensuring that decisions take into account the wider good of society. User involvement is motivated more by self-interest; aiming to improve services and health outcomes and ensuring that the view of specific user groups are taken into account (Coulter, 2006; see Figure 33.2).

user involvement and influence

Why encourage patient and public involvement?

Patients

To ensure appropriate treatment and care

To improve health outcomes

To reduce risk factors and prevent ill-health

To improve safety

To reduce complaints and litigation

Citizens

To improve service design

To determine priorities for commissioning

To manage demand

To meet expectations

To strengthen accountability

Figure 33.2 *Distinctions between patient and public involvement in health (Source: Coulter, 2006)*

Health has been an expert-dominated field. Hence user involvement has been controversial and resisted by some professionals. Involvement requires communication skills which have not traditionally been part of healthcare professionals' training. It requires equally heard voices, agreeable interactions, tolerance, and a 'give and take' attitude to get parties involved in co-ordinated actions related to policy, service, research and evaluation (El Ansari and Phillips, 2001b). Despite these challenges, the momentum for user involvement has increased.

Drivers of User Involvement

Decrease in deference – The professionals' monopoly on health related information are disappearing. Patients now have access to the Internet, challenge professionals and participate in treatment decisions.

- *Need for legitimacy* – Public scandals linked to healthcare have decreased the legitimacy of healthcare decision-making in the public eye. Involvement enhances transparency and accountability of healthcare organisations.

- *Winning hearts and minds* – The challenges that face healthcare (e.g. the increase in diabetes, lifestyle-related cancers, obesity) are ones that cannot be solved by top-down health interventions. Without the active co-operation of patients, treatment regimes are likely to be ineffective. Involvement creates ownership/commitment from patients as well as reduced costs for health providers.
- *Consumerism* – Increasingly patients are treated as consumers of health services, and concepts such as choice and satisfaction are becoming more important. Without involvement it is hard to make services responsive to patient needs.
- *Rights* – Involvement is linked to the concepts of rights and voice. People with long-term illnesses or disabilities have the right to a say in treatment decisions. This challenges the power relationships between patients and professionals (Hasler, 2006).

Reality of user involvement

Much user involvement has fallen short of the rhetoric. The power handed over to patients and the public has been limited. Gaps between the power bases of patients and professionals will need to be bridged (El Ansari et al., 2002). Most people get involved in order to make a difference, so such findings are worrying for long-term user involvement (Involve, 2005).

Some clinicians perceive the demand for involvement to be driven from the top whilst most patients are happy for their doctor to make crucial decisions. However, the demand for influence depends on circumstances, with certain decisions more likely to be deferred to professionals than others. Not all users are equally equipped to be involved. Interventions to build the capacity, information and health literacy of user groups are vital to making meaningful choices.

Evidence

Few comparative studies on the outcomes of involvement have been published. Although there are only a few robust studies of the impacts of involvement, the evidence suggests that it can provide tangible benefits. Some studies have shown reductions in the number of visits to health professionals as a result of involvement (Barlow et al., 2000), improvements in health and adoption of healthy behaviours, or increased community input in healthcare reforms (El Ansari, 2003).

Collective user involvement

User influence channelled through charities and independent patient groups is sometimes overlooked as a way of influencing health policy on behalf of users. A UK example is the use of the media by patient groups to influence decisions (e.g. the decision by the National Institute for Health and Clinical Excellence on whether or not to recommend the use of the medicine Herceptin for early cases of breast cancer).

Increasingly service provision is being contracted out to organisations in the community and voluntary sector. User involvement helps organisations to maintain their role as legitimate representatives of patient voice. The influence of patient groups is a vital counterweight to the power of hospitals/clinicians, although this role of holding health providers accountable is becoming neglected as voluntary organisations grow more dependent on income from delivering services to the public sector. Conversely, the varied size and influence of different groups mean that certain patient groups might benefit more. There might also be links between certain health charities and pharmaceutical companies.

CASE STUDY

The Expert Patients Programme (EPP) is a not for profit initiative in the UK linked to the National Health Service. The EPP provides training for people with long-term chronic conditions to help them develop new skills to manage their condition better. EPP was set up in 2002, and about 1,400 people with long-term chronic conditions (e.g. diabetes or arthritis) have been trained as Expert Patient tutors and deliver training to others who are newly diagnosed with such conditions. The aim is to help patients partner with healthcare professionals, feel confident and in control of their lives, and improve their ability to manage their condition. The impact includes gains in self-efficacy and psychological wellbeing; improvements in quality of life; and some reductions in costs of hospital use (Kennedy et al., 2007).

CONCLUSION

User involvement has been emphasised in health policy debates and practice. Widespread support for user involvement masks contradictory tendencies and latent conflict between involvement as an empowering right for patients in their relationship with professionals, and involvement as a means of achieving efficiencies and improved health outcomes.

Trends in society are driving increased user involvement, including the consumerisation of public services, a decrease in deference to figures of authority, the 'rights agenda' and the increase in complex chronic conditions. This means that despite the challenges to genuine involvement, user involvement in healthcare will continue to rise in the future.

Involvement marks a shift in medical, health and social care practice. One challenge is making engagement worthwhile for all involved while supporting patients and professionals to build their capacity to involve and be involved. The evidence base for the benefits of user involvement is lacking, as the benefits are often intangible, and hard to measure and attribute to one cause. However, involvement can lead to positive health outcomes, increased empowerment and life quality, greater satisfaction with services, improved public legitimacy of decisions, and lower healthcare costs.

FURTHER READING

Department of Health (2006) *The Expert Patients Programme*. London: Department of Health.

Involve (2005) *People and Participation: How to Put Citizens at the Heart of Decision-making*. London: Involve.

34 Collaborative and Partnership Working

Walid El Ansari

DEFINITION

The terms 'partnership' and 'coalition' are frequently used interchangeably to indicate the process by which stakeholders invest themselves with ideas, experiences and skills that collectively bear upon problems through joint decision-making and action (MUCPP, 1995).

Community partnerships (CPs) are participatory ways of mobilising community and other stakeholders to collectively address complex, long-standing health and social disparities, as partners pool their financial, material, technical and human resources (Hallfors et al., 2002; Wynn et al., 2006). Partnering is the notion of collective actions by individuals or their organisations to achieve a **more shared** communal benefit than each could accomplish as an individual player (El Ansari et al., 2001).

KEY POINTS

- Partnerships are popular components of a range of public health strategies.
- Partnership building and maintenance comprise many varied ingredients.
- The partnership 'Black Box' includes personnel, organisational, power-related and other factors.
- The challenges are difficult, but partnerships have many benefits and can be rewarding.

DISCUSSION

Partnership and collaboration between health service providers and communities have emerged as popular components of many public health strategies. Private agencies and public health organisations utilise CPs as important vehicles in generating community-based solutions to health problems. Globally, as healthcare systems face increasing demands for limited healthcare resources, collaboration and partnership are often drawn upon (Zakocs and Edwards, 2006).

Collaboration between different stakeholders in health has the advantage of synergy (Weiss et al., 2002). For instance, globally, within the HIV/AIDS arena, working in partnership has received strong recognition and joint efforts at global level in response to the epidemic (Goede and El Ansari, 2003). Similarly, within countries, district and local councils, health and social care service providers, community leaders, church and faith-based NGOs, community workers, volunteers and lay people in villages are involved together in different collaborative efforts for better HIV/AIDS prevention, care and treatment access for their communities and parishes.

The intentions of joint working arrangements are legitimate and for the greater public good. They increase citizen participation and community ownership of programmes among many vulnerable groups, including marginalised and disempowered people who previously had few participation opportunities (El Ansari and Phillips, 2001a). Further, new approaches to health and healthcare, based on multi-disciplinary and whole systems considerations, have encouraged partnership working. Health is now everyone's business: not its narrow depiction as the responsibility of the health services but a broader web of inter-sectoral, collaborative, synchronised and synergistic initiatives. Thus manpower, facilities, services and information shortages and environmental pressures all provide impetus for partnership working. Despite the appeal and promise of this approach, the factors that influence effectiveness of CPs, as well as the skills required by the partners to interact and implement a range of projects, frequently do not receive enough attention (El Ansari and Phillips, 2001b).

Partnering: the 'Black Box'

The transition of groups and partners from initial good intentions of working together, to the actual day-to-day interactions of a CP leaves a vacuum, a 'Black Box' that needs to be demystified. Collaboration is intended to facilitate parts of systems or separate systems working together towards shared and agreed goals. For diverse partners involved in joint work, CPs are more like 'living together' than marriage: it requires distinct sets of ingredients if it is to be and remain successful. The effective implementation and maintenance of CP effort needs motivated and involved people with the skills and capacity to participate in order to operate an effective climate conducive to collaboration. Thus for systemising and understanding the features that lead to short- and long-term impacts on communities, we need to answer a range of questions, for example, why do people participate? How can their collaboration be enhanced? What are the beneficial organisational/management features? Are there any historical power disparities or dominance issues that could militate against a partnership premised on equal partners (El Ansari et al., 2002)? Box 34.1 depicts the ingredients required for the process.

Box 34.1 Partnership working for public health: the essential ingredients

Personnel Factors and Barriers: Expertise, experience, operational understanding, benefits, costs, benefit/cost ratio, sense of ownership, role consensus, priorities, satisfaction, availability, turnover.

Organisational Factors and Barriers: Rules and procedures, representation, information flow, communication quality and mechanisms, interaction decision making, management capabilities, leadership capabilities, competing priorities, goal setting and decision-making, communication, leadership, stakeholder differences, lack of participation.

Power-Related Factors: Power disparities, culture of the agencies, vision, accountability, transparency, change management, group dynamics and interaction, tensions.

Other Factors: Scope of partnership, number of partners, number of problems, simple language, delays, funding cycles, sustainability, human factors, personal traits, motivation.

(*adapted from El Ansari and Phillips, 2001a*)

The basic premise is that this blend of personnel attributes, organisational features, power-related aspects as well as a range of other factors interact to generate a set of 'intermediary' variables. These intermediaries include satisfaction, commitment and a sense of ownership, outcomes and effectiveness, as well as a range of activities whether interventional, educational or preventative (Lachance et al., 2006). As the central concern for any partnership is the production of the desired outcomes, these sets of intermediary variables are sometimes employed as proxies for the accomplishment and impact of the partnership on the issue/s that it is tackling, whether service provision, prevention, care or treatment interventions.

CASE STUDY

In a study undertaken in South Africa (El Ansari et al., 2004), **these factors were mobilised** in order to identify and explore those that explained the successes of the partners. The stakeholders were the academic medical/nursing training institutions; the health services; and the lay communities, civil society and civic organisations. These CPs had the same mandate, were funded by the same donor body and had been set up in various provinces, in rural, urban and peri-urban localities. For all the parties involved, the focus was on educational competencies, partnership fostering expertise, change agents' abilities, community involvement skills, and strategic and management capacities. Hence there was interdisciplinary education for health and allied health professions as well as community development, with the aim of shifting the emphasis and resources from tertiary to secondary and primary care.

The CPs' outcomes were to enhance the skills of the health workers and the communities. They included community-based health personnel education programmes for future health professionals, and educational and reorientation programmes for health service personnel to empower them with appropriate skills and knowledge. The aims were to enhance the health of previously underprivileged communities, increasing their inputs in healthcare reforms and in the education of health professionals, as well as managing the changes. For the people, the causes of poor health were the unavailability and/or inaccessibility of health services, the insensitivity of healthcare personnel, adult illiteracy and poverty, as well as the lack of clean water and housing, poor sanitation, and the lack of early learning opportunities.

The critical dimensions

Some of the dimensions that played critical roles in the fostering of the South African CPs were:

- expertise of the professional partners;
- community members;
- sense of ownership;
- organisational and personnel barriers.

The stakeholders' expertise and skills in partnership work occupied centre stage. CPs required a distinct set of competencies that embrace educational competencies, partnership fostering expertise, community involvement skills, change agents proficiencies, and strategic and management capacities (El Ansari et al., 2002). It also included leadership skills, negotiation, networking, community organising and resource mobilization (Alexander et al., 2006).

Sense of ownership has to do with commitment to the CP's work, and a sense of pride in what it accomplishes. Partnerships are advocated as a means of increasing involvement and ownership among underprivileged constituencies. A communal sense of ownership is generated when equal agencies are collectively involved in the ground floor formation of the partnership.

The organisational barriers embraced those imposed by competing priorities among partners, differences in partners' philosophies, agency structures/systems and leadership, as well as a lack of co-ordination among partners. Similarly, personnel barriers included the expertise, priorities and turnover of members. Recruiting/retaining members in a collaborative effort is often a difficult task.

CONCLUSION

There is little doubt that effective partnerships between service providers and communities will be the single most important governance innovation in the coming years. The partnership approach is a very promising one, but in order for it to succeed, administrators, health workers, community members and other stakeholders will need a good understanding of the variety of intricate and intertwined factors that operate within the 'Black Box'. As CP processes engage stakeholders to bring their of ideas, experiences and skills collectively to bear on the problem through mechanisms for joint decision-making and action, the melange of aspects and facets of partnership fostering need to be demystified for those who are involved. I hope this contribution will play a role in increasing the transparency of the type of connections, processes, interactions, contingencies and exchanges that are the essential ingredients making partnership work effective and efficient.

FURTHER READING

El Ansari, W., Phillips, C. J., and Hammick, M. (2001) 'Collaboration and partnerships: developing the evidence base', *Health and Social Care in the Community*, 9(4): 215–27.

El Ansari, W., Phillips, C. J. and Zwi, A. B. (2004) 'Collaboration in health: public health nurses' perspectives', *Public Health Nursing*, 21(3): 278–87.

35 Evidence-based Practice

Gail Louw

DEFINITION

One of the earliest and certainly the most influential definitions of evidence-based practice (EBP) is by Sackett et al. (1996): 'Evidence-based medicine is the conscientious, explicit and judicious use of current best evidence in making decisions about the care of individual patients.' The focus of this definition is clearly on the use of research to inform decision-makers and enhance their decision-making capabilities. The decision-makers appear here to be the clinicians, those responsible for the care of individual patients, and indeed the experience and judgement of clinicians is an integral part of the process. However, an unrepresented group in this definition are patients, users or clients and it is essential that their subjective values, preferences, beliefs and opinions are incorporated into the decision-making process.

KEY POINTS

- The philosophical change underpinning EBP is a move from expert opinion, from an entrenched approach of doing what has always been done, to accessing evidence and using it, together with clinical judgement and patient opinion, to inform care.
- This philosophical change is a response to: variations in clinical practice, exponential increase in evidence and the need to keep up to date with the evidence, the inadequacies of relying on traditional reviews of the literature and the increased expectation of openness and involvement of public, patients and users.
- The processes for undertaking EBP are to: produce a research question, search and appraise the evidence, select and option, implement it and evaluate performance.

DISCUSSION

The exponential growth and impact of EBP has been an almost unprecedented phenomenon (Trinder and Reynolds, 2000). EBP is the cornerstone of current health policy and has been instrumental in acting as a model for similar developments in other disciplines: evidence-based education (Davies, 1999), evidence-based social work (e.g. *Journal of Evidence Based Social Work*), and evidence-based information systems (Atkins and Louw, 2000) to name just a few. It has also precipitated the introduction of numerous new journals (e.g. *Evidence Based Nursing* and *Evidence Based Mental Health*), evidence-based bulletins (such as Bandolier, and the pre-eminent source of good quality research, the Cochrane Library – http://www.cochrane.org/).

EBP has become fundamental in the research and practice of healthcare because it meets the needs of providers, consumers and commissioners to influence care. Every healthcare consumer or practitioner is in a position to assess the quality of research evidence and establish for themselves the effectiveness of particular interventions (Sackett and Parkes, 1998; Bandolier, 2000; MacRae et al., 2004), and thus participate in their own decision-making about healthcare provision (Gray, 2004).

Asking a question

A fundamental skill needed to practise EBP is to be able to ask a focused research question. A useful framework exists for this purpose, and it is worth attempting to use this framework for any kind of question, therapy, exposure to disease, diagnostic test, prognostic factor, risk factors, treatment or perceptions. The framework is known as PICO: Population (or Patient), Intervention, Comparison and Outcome, and the Comparison component is optional (see Table 35.1).

Searching for the evidence

It is possible to undertake either an extensive search or 'quick and dirty' searches. The type is dependent on the purpose of the search and undertaking a systematic review will require a more elaborate and far-reaching search than would be necessary to answer an immediate question about a specific patient query.

The Cochrane Library provides excellent quality evidence and should therefore be the first area to search as well as evidence-based sources such as Bandolier. Other key areas to search are: electronic databases

Table 35.1 *Examples of the PICO framework for asking a focused question*

	Population	Intervention	Comparison	Outcome
Example 1: RCT of a therapy	Amongst adults wishing to give up smoking	do nicotine replacement patches given by a GP	compared to nicotine replacement patches given by a specialist smoking cessation adviser	lead to higher quit rates?
Example 2: Qualitative study	How do pregnant women	who are offered HIV tests		feel?
Example 3: Prognosis observational study. (Must be prospective as it would be difficult to establish the accuracy of the alcohol intake)	Amongst people who are diagnosed as hepatitis C positive	what level of alcohol intake		increases the risk of cirrhosis of the liver?
Example 4: Diagnostic test	Amongst females at risk of chlamydia,	does an endo-cervical swab	compared to a PCR urine test	produce the same number of true positives and true negatives?

(such as Medline, PubMed, Cinahl, Psychlit), grey literature (conference proceedings and theses, accessible via electronic databases such as Sigle or Zetoc), references of references and contacting authors (to find out if they know of any studies that have been undertaken but not published, possibly as a result of publication bias – the problems of studies with negative outcomes not being published: Dickersin and Min, 1993).

Levels of evidence

There are a number of 'hierarchies of evidence' and many are remarkably similar. Most omit any reference to qualitative studies, which is unfortunate as it negates the importance of these works and reinforces

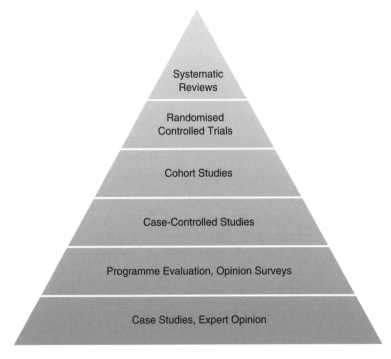

Figure 35.1 *Pyramid of evidence – quantitative studies*

the conviction amongst many that they are second best. However, it is inappropriate to combine quantitative and qualitative studies in one hierarchy. For this reason two hierarchies are presented here. Figure 35.1 is a hierarchy of evidence from quantitative studies while Figure 35.2 from Salmond's (2007) 'pyramid of evidence' is based on evidence from experience. In this instance, qualitative studies are valued and evidence from quantitative studies is considered less significant.

Appraising the evidence

There is a useful definition of critical appraisal which at first glance seems an unachievable task for those who are not research literate. 'Critical appraisal is the process of systematically examining research evidence to assess its validity, results and relevance before using it to inform a decision' (Hill and Spittlehouse, 2003). However, there are many checklists which provide the assistance that enables people with

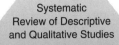

Systematic
Review of Descriptive
and Qualitative Studies

Evidence From a Single Descriptive
or Qualitative Study

Expert Opinion, Expert Communities

Evidence Based on Quantitative Approaches

Figure 35.2 *Pyramid of evidence – description of experience (Source: Salmond, 2007)*

only the slightest initiation of research methods to critically appraise a research study. The checklists are specific to different types of study and are available from (as examples) Greenhalgh (2006), Crombie (1996), and numerous websites (e.g. http://www.sign.ac.uk/guidelines/fulltext/50/annexc.html; http://www.shef.ac.uk/scharr/ir/units/critapp/index.htm).

Systematic reviews

The quantity of research papers is as extensive as their quality. Assessing the quality of one paper does not establish certainty of evidence, even where the standard is acceptable, simply because there may be other papers with the same research question which reach different conclusions. The proliferation of papers and journals is overwhelming (Davidoff et al., 1995). Neither practitioners, undertaking normal work activities, nor patients/consumers can be expected to read, appraise and amalgamate all the existing studies in the world literature on a specific research question.

It is for this reason that systematic reviews have become so prolific. Over ten years, the number of systematic reviews has grown to the extent that there are around 5,000 completed systematic reviews, all of which have gone through extensive and rigorous review procedures, within the

Cochrane Library Database of Systematic Reviews. Systematic reviews meet the need of finding, appraising and amalgamating all studies that look at a specific question in either published or unpublished format in any language (Centre for Reviews and Dissemination, 2001). The resulting single publication presents a clear search strategy: a list of all included studies which reach a pre-established quality standard, justification for all excluded studies, and some form of synthesis of all the data, either as a meta-analysis or a narrative, with a final 'bottom line' conclusion.

Good systematic reviews of randomised controlled trials are regarded as being at the apex of the hierarchy of evidence (Greenhalgh, 2006). Findings from these systematic reviews take precedence over all other single studies, though some regard large randomised controlled trials as of equal value. The weight that systematic reviews carry therefore places a responsibility on the author or team of authors to produce a piece of research that is exceptional in its rigour and minimisation of bias.

Implementation and evaluation

As with all projects which are undertaken rigorously, implementing, disseminating and evaluating the processes and outcomes at different points of follow-up are essential.

CASE STUDY

An important public health problem that emerged in recent years was the fear amongst some parents that providing their children with the MMR vaccination would result in Crohn's disease or autism. This well known phenomenon was the result of a study published in the *Lancet* by Wakefield et al. (1998).

There is a wealth of discussion about this paper, and entering MMR into Google is sufficient to identify a whole range of sources for further deliberation, including statistics, and articles that refute or support the facts. How can one assess which articles or opinion pieces are valid? The answer is that critical appraisal skills enable the reader to assess validity. In this case, much of the work is already done, and a response by Professor Trish Greenhalgh goes through a critical appraisal checklist with responses (http://briandeer.com/mmr/lancet-greenhalgh.htm).

FURTHER READING

Guyatt, G. and Rennie, D. (eds) (2002) *Users' Guides to the Medical Literature: A Manual for Evidence-based Clinical Practice*. Chigaco: AMA Press.

Rycroft-Malone, J. et al. (2004) 'What counts as evidence in evidence-based practice', *Journal of Advanced Nursing*, 47(1): 81–90.

36 Public Health and Contemporary Health Issues

Mike Thomas

DEFINITION

The concept of contemporary is generally used to convey what is present and current in society. In some settings it is used to describe being in fashion, up to date and modern, others mean something co-existing with another. One could argue that all three applications occur in the public health arena. For example socio-economic inequalities in health have remained current in the UK despite a rise in relative living standards, dietary fads come and go in short bursts of lifestyle fashion, whilst infectious diseases and virus-carrying hosts coexist with society despite great strides in pharmaceutical therapies.

Defining contemporary public health issues is therefore open to interpretation and the focus can alter over a short time. This problem has bedevilled public health policy for nearly 200 years. More recently, Ashton and Seymour (1992) stressed that the health environment is not just the physical world but also the psychological and social worlds. A few years earlier Rowland and Cooper (1983) argued that the physical world (housing, the work environment, clean air, water and food) had a strong relationship with population health yet it was of equal importance to individual habits and lifestyle choices such as nicotine, alcohol and dietary intake.

KEY POINTS

- Contemporary health issues can mean new public health concerns but also revisiting historically persistent issues.
- Contemporary health issues may refer to fashionable lifestyles.
- Public health research has influenced health and social care policy since the early eighteenth century, but sometimes has had less success in gaining resources for specific public health concerns.
- There are a number of sub-specialities within public health that have a common theme of prevention and health promotion.

DISCUSSION

How to raise the profile of illness prevention and health promotion on a societal scale is an essential skill requirement for anyone working in public health. It is no surprise that the increasing number of sub-specialities has led to competing agendas for those charged with prioritising healthcare resources. There is a large body of evidence going back nearly 300 years which demonstrates the links between good health, environmental factors, inequalities in income, familial influences, gender, education and lifestyle choices. McKeown's (1976) work demonstrated that from the early nineteenth century until the implementation of immunisation programmes the major cause of reduced mortality in the UK population was improved standards in water, housing, food and waste disposal. The Victorian age responded to such clear correlations with a range of social and engineering interventions. Still it took nearly two more centuries before issues of equality related to gender, sex and race became enshrined in the legal system.

The development of public health in the UK shows a striking difference between the social and medical advances and the improvements for certain aspects of wellbeing. Ashton and Seymour (1992) point out that those with societal power had a vested interest in preventing infectious diseases, as anything that could pass through the population as a whole would inevitably strike them and their families. This may, in part, explain the United States' historical intervention in immunisation programmes and the lack of response to other agendas which have a less negative impact on the elite. Certainly the early part of the twentieth century saw an increase in both political and legislative activities around hospital-based care which culminated in the Beveridge Report (DHSS, 1942) and the subsequent birth of the National Health Service (1945–48). The state had moved towards full control of health resources and within a few years the Department of Health focused on treatment strategies whilst other public health areas such as housing, employment, environmental health, energy sources, transport and food production were scattered across a number of ministries.

The paradox identified by many in public health then arose. It is known that contemporary issues such as cancer, cardiovascular disease, depression, obesity, drug and alcohol abuse, sexually transmitted diseases, more acute problems (injuries, accidents, viral outbreaks) and the confirmed threats to health caused by climate change cannot be tackled by an illness-focused health service. The positive effects of a good education, income, family life, leisure pursuits, transport, environmental recycling, reusable energy, and the geography of where we live and how we live directly impact on promotion of good health. The paradox is that policies aimed at improving health have concentrated more on expanding healthcare services and less on interdisciplinary community services, with the result that resources have been spent on treating conditions that were preventable in the first place (Ashton and Seymour, 1992; Baggot, 2000; Luck et al., 2000; Layard, 2005; Roger and Pilgrim, 2005).

This paradox has been recognised by successive UK governments. Public health increased in prominence with a recognition that contemporary issues could not be addressed by different governmental departments without a co-ordinated lead. In Thatcher's government the major issues of the day were HIV/AIDS, drug abuse and cardiovascular disease. Even here there was a paradox, as the government refused to support any national census of the sexual habits of the populace (Thomas and Hynes, 1998).

Nevertheless the Conservatives were not successful at co-ordinating inter-departmental working. In fact there was a proliferation of specialists and consultants, advisers and committees competing for scarce resources in a government whose philosophy was to cut public spending. Once again the public health paradox was observed. Screening identified those individuals who required treatment, but little emphasis was placed on prevention. Interventions to deal with lifestyle issues were discouraged and so more resource pressure was placed on an illness-orientated NHS.

The Conservatives did introduce *Promoting Better Health* (DHSS, 1987) and *Community Care: Agenda for Action* (DHSS, 1988) policies which introduced economic incentives for GPs who carried out health promotion. They also introduced new management practices such as fees for ophthalmic and dental treatments which were heavily criticised at the time. The objective was to encourage less reliance on the state and provide more choice through the 'consumer' model of health delivery. By 1994 the Commission for Social Justice found that economic inequality in the UK had deteriorated to pre-war levels, with a greater number of the population surviving on less than half the average income while homelessness doubled. Rejecting repeated calls for departmental co-ordination (Acheson Report, 1998) it was not until 1992 that the *Health of the Nation* policy paper was published which had a stronger public health emphasis and gave targets for the issues of the time.

The growing body of evidence produced in specialist fields within a previously fragmented public health approach led to a rejection of Thatcher's pro-market approach and provided guidance to the new Labour government as older public health issues began to re-emerge alongside new ones. What is clear is that public health gained prominence in the policies of all main political parties. Consequently in 1997 Blair committed his party to confront public health issues by focusing on the social and economic basis of ill health.

A decade later contemporary issues remain the continuous fight against coexisting diseases such as hospital-based infections, the rise in sexually transmitted infections, seasonal outbreaks and food-sourced outbreaks. A growing area of multidisciplinary activity is around the co-ordination of health and sustainable development in response to climate change. The introduction of policies for the Primary Care Trusts, the ban on smoking in public places, cervical vaccinations for young females, and closer governmental co-ordination of approaches to cancer, cardiac disease, mental health, economic inequality and educational targets indicate that contemporary issues remain the management of recurring problems and pathogenic entities and tackling the present threat of climate change.

CASE STUDY

Sustainable development is an objective for the local authority, and the council is charged with producing a Local Action Plan. The council realises that to meet targets it has to include the Primary Care Trust, the local hospital, voluntary organisations, schools, local people and various council departments. It is concerned about 'committee' fatigue, over-stretching resources and disengaging the population from decision-making.

A council-sponsored open forum was planned, with a number of key speakers who were identified as experts in conveying local public health issues. This forum showed that small projects supported by Local Area Agreements, and PCT funding would be the most appropriate way forward. Projects included waste management; a parent/guardian information drive regarding immunisation; a well man and well woman clinic delivered in and around the town centre for local employers; a nutrition and exercise toolkit for local schools, and the supply of low energy light bulbs to all households agreeing to participate in a free energy audit.

There was initial resistance and a low participation in two of the projects but the rest were successful in reaching targets. Other local authorities and central government departments became interested in the process of implementation and the resulting publicity led to more resources being given to further collaborative projects.

CONCLUSION

By the turn of this century public health had risen to the top of the political health agenda and the field had developed into sub-specialisms such as occupational health, families, gender issues, mental health and policy. Recently there has been more emphasis on sustainable developments in response to climate change, on nutrition and exercise, on population growth and the potential impact on infrastructure, on user involvement in healthcare and a return to an old theme of controlling contagious diseases and infections.

Contemporary health issues can therefore mean something new and current (climate change); fashionable and modern (the growth in individual therapies, the concentration on image and self-presentation) and revisiting enduring public health concerns about disease control, economic inequity and lifestyle choices.

FURTHER READING

Layard, R. (2005) *Happiness – Lessons from a New Science*. London: Penguin.

UK Public Health Association (2007) *Climates and Change – The Urgent Need to Connect Health and Sustainable Development*. London: UKPHA.

public health and contemporary health

37 Public Health and Physical Activity

Hayley Mills, Diane Crone and Walid El Ansari

DEFINITION

There has been a proliferation of physical activity included in public health policies in the last decade (DH, 1999, 2004a; DCMS/Strategy Unit, 2002) and an evidence-based practice in physical activity promotion within primary care has emerged (Crone et al., 2004). The most common programmes available are Physical Activity Referral Schemes (PARS). Such schemes involve the referral of primary care patients by a health professional (usually GP or nurse) to an exercise provider for a programme of supervised physical activity normally within a leisure centre setting (Crone et al., 2004).

KEY POINTS

- The PARS scheme improves confidence, motivation, wellbeing and knowledge of physical activity.
- It has social benefits – confidence, enjoyment and satisfaction.
- Physiological measures demonstrate significant positive changes which if sustained may lead to health benefits.
- Retired people have exhibited the highest success rate.
- The facilitator's role is pivotal in providing support and motivation.

DISCUSSION

As the emphasis on promoting physical activity in primary care has developed, the number of PARS in operation increased rapidly from 157 reported schemes in 1994, to more than 800 across the UK in 2004 (Labour Research Department, 2004). Recent estimations indicate as many as 1,300 schemes nationwide (Mental Health Foundation,

2005). Despite the abundance of PARS across the country there is a continuing lack of robust evidence regarding effectiveness (Hillsdon et al., 2004).

In measuring a scheme's success, researchers have been restricted to poor quality or inadequate data. As a consequence the success of a PARS is often measured merely by its attendance levels (the number of participants who commence, drop out or successfully complete the scheme) (Wright Foundation Conference, 2003). This excludes issues of quality such as the experiences. Holistic health evaluations should incorporate patients' opinions along with health and adherence measures (Dugdill et al., 2005). The National Quality Assurance Framework (NQAF) highlights this need for rigorous evaluation that incorporates qualitative methods (DH, 2001a).

CASE STUDY: HEALTHWISE – A PARS, BASED IN GREENWICH, LONDON

Healthwise is a partnership project between Greenwich Leisure Limited (GLL), Greenwich Teaching Primary Care Trust (GTPCT) and Greenwich Council. Government funding in the form of Single Regeneration Budget funding was used to develop this PARS across GLL leisure centres in the London Borough of Greenwich. The scheme commenced in January 2005 and utilised five leisure centres for exercise options such as gym-based supervised sessions, circuit training, water-based aerobics and exercise to music sessions. A facilitator was assigned to the patients to assess and oversee their progression. The scheme was provided at a subsidised rate to the referred patients. Its duration was 12 to 26 weeks, depending on the patient's progress. The primary aim of the Healthwise scheme was to ensure that affordable and accessible opportunities were provided for people to become more physically active in order to improve the health and wellbeing of the Greenwich population and to reduce health inequalities.

The evaluation covered the duration of the Healthwise project from January 2005 to March 2007. It incorporated an action research element to provide best practice guidance in order to ensure the programme was continually developed. Feedback was given on a quarterly basis to the steering group, providing interim conclusions and recommendations regarding the scheme's progress, which were acted upon where appropriate.

A mixed method approach to the evaluation of Healthwise comprised quantitative and qualitative methods that were employed through three distinct but complementary phases. The quantitative methods included data routinely collected such as patients' age, gender, ethnicity, occupation, attendance, referral reason, along with pre and post measures of weight, wellbeing (sf-12), systolic and diastolic blood pressure. In parallel, the qualitative component included descriptive observation, focus groups and interviews. Hence adequate quantitative data to assess the scope of the scheme coupled with qualitative data to determine the depth of change for the individual was collected (Clark and McLeroy, 1998).

The qualitative data comprised four focus groups with a total of 17 patients (13 women and 4 men); individual telephone interviews with seven referrers (two doctors and five nurses); and individual face-to-face interviews with the four facilitators of the scheme. The findings highlighted the social benefits that were perceived by the patients. Patients also demonstrated potential outcomes such as confidence, enjoyment and satisfaction. The connection between enjoyment and adherence has also been supported by research (Wankel, 1993). Furthermore patients expressed an increased awareness and knowledge of health behaviour: 'Well I would still carry on, I think I know enough about it now to do that.' Potentially a valuable finding, this may help to establish long-term behaviour change. The social aspect is also deemed by the facilitators as important to the patient: 'They come for the interaction a little more than they come for the exercise.' The finding that that the social aspect of physical activity can be motivating is supported by Eyler et al. (1997).

A further notable finding was the importance facilitators placed on the patient's readiness to change. The findings also pointed to the significance of the facilitator's role in providing support and motivation, as exemplified by a facilitator who reported: '…a lot of them like to feel cared about, don't they, like someone is actually taking an interest in them'. Facilitators were trained in the principles of motivational interviewing and as such were aware of these issues and acknowledged them as influential factors for patients. Referrers (health professionals) further complimented the low cost of the scheme and its accessibility to patients on low incomes.

The quantitative component of the evaluation of Healthwise consisted of 1,315 complete data records. Patients who reached the end of the scheme and attended their final assessment were categorised as successful. A 57 per cent success rate was recorded, which is encouraging in comparison with previous research where completion rates for schemes ranged from 14 to 56 per cent (Hammond et al., 1997; Stephens, 1998; Taylor et al., 1998).

A comparison of those attending the scheme and the Greenwich population as a whole showed an effective targeting of ethnic groups. This effective targeting continued, with a large percentage of both unemployed and retired patients taking part in the scheme. This is important, as the health-damaging behaviour of inactivity is not distributed equally across the population (DH, 2003a). Certain population groups tend to be less active than others and it is often these same groups that report the poorest health (DH, 2003a). Inequalities have been observed, with poor health in the lower socio-economic groups (Wagstaff, 2002). Interventions like PARS might need to target these sections of the community and therefore can potentially play a role in reducing health inequalities.

Furthermore, with PARS the retired section of the community achieved the highest success, with a completion rate of 59.1 per cent and lowest failure rate of 32.9 per cent. The percentage of success improved with age, showing a steady increase up to 85 years old. This is a positive finding particularly in the light of the Greenwich borough statistics which indicate that only 7.5 per cent of the over-55-year-olds are physically active (three 30-minute exercise sessions per week). Referral to the Healthwise scheme is most common for pre-existing health conditions such as cardiovascular disease (17.5 per cent), metabolic (36.3 per cent) and orthopaedic diseases (24.7 per cent), whose outcomes may be modified by regular exercise.

Statistically significant differences in body weight ($p < 0.001$) and mean arterial pressure ($p < 0.01$) were found before and after participation in the scheme. As these statistically significant reductions were small, the individual health benefits that could accumulate from these changes might be questionable. However, the changes were in the positive direction and health benefits may arise if the health behaviour change could be sustained in the longer term. Furthermore, a small reduction in blood pressure leading to a reduction in the risk of consequent ischaemic heart disease could result in potentially significant savings to the NHS (NICE, 2006). This demonstrates the potential value of such schemes for the population as a whole. A preventative measure of this nature may benefit the population although seemingly offering only a small benefit, particularly in the short term to the individual. The lack of immediate or substantial health rewards for the individual may begin to explain why interventions can appear problematic for patients to adhere to. Stronger individual motivators in this case were provided from the more immediate enhanced self-esteem and social inclusion, rather than the more distant health rewards.

In order to provide information on wellbeing outcomes of the scheme, the Short Form 12 version 2 (SF–12®) Health Survey was administered to 116 scheme participants, at two points: on commencement and completion of the scheme. Statistically significant differences from baseline were observed at the post measure for six of the eight outcomes and for the physical component summary score. The findings from the SF–12 indicated that successful participation in the Healthwise PARS positively affected patients' wellbeing, particularly the SF–12 wellbeing components of general health, bodily pain, physical functioning and vitality.

CONCLUSION

Healthwise has successfully targeted patients among those at risk from health inequalities, providing a valuable service to the more deprived sections of the community. Qualitative research revealed the importance of the experience to the patients, who gained valuable benefits such as improved confidence, motivation, wellbeing and knowledge of physical activity.

Collectively, these findings demonstrate the potential role that PARS can play in enhancing the holistic health of individuals.

FURTHER READING

Hillsdon, M., Foster, C., Naidoo, B. and Crombie, H. (2004) *The Effectiveness of Public Health Interventions for Increasing Physical Activity among Adults: A Review of Reviews*. London: Department of Health.

The Mental Health Foundation (2005) *Up and Running: Exercise Therapy and the Treatment of Mild or Moderate Depression in Primary Care*. London: The Mental Health Foundation.

38 Public Health and Nutrition

Basma Ellahi

DEFINITION

The Nutrition Society defines public health nutrition as the science and art of preventing disease, prolonging life and promoting health through the medium of sustainable and equitable improvements in the food and nutrition system (Buss, 1998; Nutrition Society, 2007). The contribution of nutrition to the public health approach to prevention of the burden of diseases (non-communicable and chronic) as well as to promoting health and wellbeing and prolonging life is undisputable. A thorough knowledge of nutrition and the body's nutritional requirements and psychosocial aspects of food habits and choice throughout the lifespan is now recognised as an essential defined public health specialism (Nutrition Society, 2007).

KEY POINTS

- A balanced diet is important for good health.
- Nutritional requirements vary across the lifespan and are greatest during rapid growth phases.
- Nutritional standards provide a yardstick for assessing the diets of populations.
- Food-based guidelines and models allow people to translate nutrition principles into practice.
- Public health nutrition focuses on the promotion of good health through primary prevention of diet-related illness.
- Public health nutrition is informed by nutritional epidemiology identifying the nature of diet–disease relationships.
- Public health nutrition relies on the principles of health promotion requiring communication skills and understanding of the influences governing the way people live and choose what to eat.

DISCUSSION

A nutritious diet provides the basis for health promotion and disease prevention, making it an important part of public health policy. Good nutrition or optimal nutrition is achieved when a person eats a varied diet containing all the nutrients in sufficient amounts as determined by dietary reference values. Essentially this enables a person to develop, to grow or to maintain the body and its stores for later use and thus allows for natural variation for health and disease prevention. Under-nutrition occurs when individuals consume fewer nutrients than the body requires, resulting in a nutritional deficit. It is most common in poverty and in those with increased nutritional requirements. In contrast over-nutrition occurs when a person consumes an excessive amount of nutrients. Significant levels of illness and mortality have been linked to dietary habits such as a low intake of fresh fruit and vegetables, fibre and the consumption of excessive amounts of energy (WHO, 2003). Higher energy intake over that utilised is the fundamental cause of overweight and obesity. The prevalence of obesity has trebled in the UK since the 1980s, to the point where now nearly two-thirds of men and over half of women are either overweight or obese (DH, 2001a). Obesity has been implicated as a risk factor in a number of diseases including diabetes, coronary heart disease (CHD), osteoarthritis, hypertension and some cancers, and is predicted to cost the NHS £3.6 billion by 2010 (DH, 2000c). This has been supported by government policies (DH, 1999, 2004b). The National Service Frameworks for Coronary Heart Disease (DH, 2000c) and Diabetes (DH, 2001d) also identify diet and nutrition key health outcomes.

To maintain healthy populations most countries have developed nutrition standards for major nutrients to act as a yardstick of adequacy when assessing diets of population groups. People eat food not nutrients so dietary guidelines provide recommendations that promote healthy eating habits. These are based on food groups such as fats, sugars, etc. but also include recommendations for physical activity. Like many countries, the UK has developed these into visual models which can be used with populations. Since not all foods fit into one category neatly the food guides emphasise the need for variety and balance, and provide a range of daily servings. The UK has recently adopted the Balance of Good Health model to the Eat Well plate (www.food.gov.uk) and the USA has adapted its food pyramid to include physical activity more overtly (www.mypyramid.usda.gov).

Nutritional epidemiology is the scientific basis upon which public health nutrition is built. It is the study of diet-related diseases in the population and is informed by a complex set of principles which enable collection of data on human nutrition and community health with a purpose or research question in mind. This enables the effect of other factors such as age, gender or smoking to be taken account of and the exposure variable and outcome measure of interest can be determined with sufficient precision to enable a reliable estimate of the relationship of interest to be addressed. This has led to our current understanding of the diet–disease relationships and many studies still continue to determine others. Over time we have learned that patterns of food consumption are as important as the influence of individual components. Evaluation of interventions also relies on epidemiological research principles and is important for assessing effectiveness (see Chapter 39, Community Food Initiatives). Thus the relevance of nutritional epidemiology to public health becomes clearer over time.

Nutritional screening and assessment of risk involves the examination of factors such as height, weight, laboratory values on biochemistry, diet, appetite, illness or diagnosis to determine the risk of nutritional problems in specific populations. Screening may target pregnant women for example on B vitamin and folate levels, the elderly on malnutrition, or those with nutritional disorders such as cardiac disorders to detect deficiencies or potential imbalances. A nutritionist, dietician or health professional may perform the screening, which can be part of a routine screen in the case of a public health nutritionist or specific to referred clients in the case of a dietician or health professional. In public health, nutrition screening can be applied to seemingly well populations to assess body mass index as an indicator of height to weight relationship and eating habits, environment, and functional status. The output from screening is a calculation of the level of risk (or risk score) for the nutritional problem. Individuals or populations at higher risk should be given a comprehensive nutritional assessment, whereas those at lower to moderate risk should be re-evaluated over a period of time.

Nutritional assessment is undertaken for individuals or populations at risk and involves a comprehensive nutritional assessment to examine additional factors and determine the extent of under- or over-nutrition. In this way a baseline assessment can be established and a diet/exercise plan developed as appropriate. At this stage a registered dietician would be involved.

Finally, public health nutrition is about solving problems and a PHN cycle has been developed to help achieve this aim:

1 Identify the key nutrition problem.
2 Set goal.
3 Define clear objectives for goal.
4 Create quantitative targets.
5 Develop programme.
6 Implement programme.
7 Evaluate programme.

Higher rates of nutrition-related disease can be found to cluster in disadvantaged groups (Acheson, 1998; Graham, 1993). Health intelligence shows that people from lower socio-economic groups suffer from higher rates of coronary heart disease, and that rates of blood pressure and stroke are higher; this is also the case for certain cancers and prevalence of dental caries in children. Also known as the health gradient, this results in effects of differences in income, housing, education and the living and working environment throughout an individual's lifetime (Gordon et al., 1999; Power et al., 1997). Key determinants include differing economic circumstances (Kennedy and Ling, 1997; Darmon et al., 2002; Burgon, 2007), nutritional knowledge and awareness (Dallongeville et al., 2003; Wardle et al., 2000), fruit and vegetable consumption (Henderson et al., 2002; De Irala-Estévez et al., 2000; Giskes et al., 2002), vitamin, mineral and trace element intake, maternal nutrition and infant feeding practices (Dubois and Girard, 2001), access to and availability of high quality nutritious food at affordable prices (Travers, 1996; Cummins and Macintyre, 2002), and the absence of basic cooking skills and confidence in food preparation (Caraher et al., 1999; Kennedy et al., 1998).

CASE STUDY: UK STRATEGY TO INCREASING FRUIT AND VEGETABLE CONSUMPTION

UK strategy on increasing fruit and vegetable consumption is a classic example of the public health nutrition approach to disease prevention that employs sustainable and equitable improvements in the food and nutrition system.

Average consumption of fruit and vegetables in England is 2.8 portions per day (DH, 2005b), which clearly falls short of the recommended five portions a day. However, this figure does not highlight the wide differences in consumption, with the lowest consumption being in children and young people, men and people in lower socio-economic groups. The government piloted a range of 5 A DAY initiatives in 5 areas across the country at the start of the decade and evaluated their success. Each area employed a range of activities, which were broadly categorised into activities to improve access and availability and activities to improve attitudes to change and develop awareness of the need for change. Strategies to increase consumption were targeted in areas of need and took into account the different influences on health. Projects to tackle access and availability included food co-ops, initiatives with local retailers and fruit and vegetable voucher schemes, allotment schemes, promotional work with supermarkets and workplace catering initiatives. Projects focusing on attitudes and awareness included targeted 5 A DAY promotional campaigns using a settings approach, e.g. in schools or nurseries, tasting sessions, improving cooking and food preparation skills through Cook and Taste programmes, nutrition education programmes and communication campaigns on a local and national level (DH, 2003a). Evaluation showed change in awareness, purchase and consumption across a range of age groups.

FURTHER READING

Buss, D. (1998) 'Registered Public Health Nutritionist (RPHNutr): a new qualification in public health nutrition', *Nutrition and Food Science*, 98(3).

Nutrition Society (2007) *Voluntary Register of Nutritionists: Guide to Registration as a Nutritionist*. Cambridge: Nutrition Society.

39 Community Food Initiatives and Public Health

Basma Ellahi

DEFINITION

Developing and establishing community-based food initiatives to improve nutrition-related health, particularly in areas of health inequalities, has received significant support in recent years. In recognition of the complex interplay of factors determining food choice (Dahlgren and Whitehead, 1991) and the limitations of traditional approaches to health campaigns community food-based initiatives have been gaining popularity as a method of directing health promotion efforts at low-income populations. The schemes aim to improve the diet of local people through increasing nutritional education and improving food-related skills, such as cooking and shopping, by utilising individuals indigenous to the local community to deliver a range of activities within the community including 'Cook and Eat' sessions and promotional events.

KEY POINTS

- Socio-economic inequalities in health are a recognised problem in the UK.
- Lower socio-economic classes suffer a greater incidence of premature and low birthweight babies, heart disease, stroke and some cancers, partly as a consequence of poor diet, which is identified as a major risk factor for many chronic diseases.
- People in lower socio-economic groups have unhealthy diets predominantly because of their social and economic circumstances, not through ignorance or irresponsible choice.

- In industrialised countries, as cost becomes an increasing constraint, energy-dense but nutrient-poor cheaper foods such as cereals, sugars and fats become more important. More expensive nutrient-dense fruits and vegetables become less important.
- In Britain the National Diet and Nutrition Survey found that men and women in households in receipt of state benefit ate significantly fewer portions of fruit and/or vegetables a day than in non-benefit households.
- The absence of cooking skills can be a barrier to widening food choice to include healthier options.
- Caraher et al. (1999) reported a strong positive association between confidence in using different cooking methods and social class.
- Confidence in using all cooking techniques was high in the upper social classes, with the exception of one method, deep fat frying, which was the cooking technique that individuals from the lowest social class were most confident in using.
- This is further supported by a study revealing that individuals with unskilled occupations were significantly more likely to own a deep fat fryer than other groups (Efstathiou et al., 2004).
- It has been suggested that this less healthy method of cooking is very popular in low socio-economic populations, contributing to their already inadequate dietary habits.

DISCUSSION

Disparities in health across socio-economic groups ensue from a combination of barriers to adopting healthy eating guidelines experienced by the lower classes relating to income, self-confidence and ability to cook, for example. Therefore addressing nutritional inequalities in these individuals could be assisted by schemes that aim to promote the selection of healthier food choices within the constraints of a small budget and facilitates these behaviour changes with enhanced self-efficacy due to greater comprehension of the association between diet and health and improved food-related skills.

Traditional nutrition education has achieved limited success in low-income groups and providing culturally sensitive and appropriate advice is fundamental, particularly for those living in disadvantaged areas (Kennedy et al., 1999). This has resulted in more public health initiatives based in the community. Furthermore, greater community involvement in identifying the needs of the community and designing the solution to be implemented instils in the community a degree of power, and in individuals a sense of empowerment (Easterling et al., 2003). Such an approach, increasing the problem-solving capabilities of individuals and organisations, is referred to as capacity building, and creates self-sustaining united communities.

Increasingly as part of a capacity-building strategy, individuals *from* the community are being recruited to deliver healthcare services *within* that community as community health workers (CHWs). The use of local people in this function recognises their natural empathy with their native community and their unique understanding of the particular difficulties and limitations experienced by residents. Consequently they serve as 'culture brokers', mediators between two cultural systems, in this case acting as the linking step between the community and healthcare systems or directly providing healthcare services themselves as peer educators. CHWs have also been employed in a variety of food-based initiatives and achieved considerable success. 'Cook and Eat' sessions have been shown to be particularly appealing to low-income groups (Buttriss et al., 2004) but can be criticised for being labour intensive and not addressing the wider issues relating to food poverty. Nevertheless, Kennedy et al. (1999) demonstrated positive behaviour changes, including changes in food purchased and cooking methods, in individuals in contact with CHWs in Bolton. Additionally the CHWs made four times as many contacts with community members compared with community dieticians, establishing their demonstrable cost-effectiveness. In particular, the CHWs accessed traditionally 'hard-to-reach' groups including the homeless, unemployed and young mothers residing in hostels. Likewise, socially disadvantaged pregnant African-American women in Mississippi, USA also responded well to peer education from CHWs, demonstrating an improvement in nutrition knowledge and dietary behaviour despite previously exhibiting poor utilisation of healthcare services (Boyd and Windsor, 2003). Moreover, the peer education approach has been shown to be successful with higher socio-economic groups too. Kunkel et al. (2004) found that peer educators providing one-to-one nutritional education was effective in improving general and sports nutrition knowledge in young female athletes. In summary, the few community food-based initiatives that have been evaluated suggest that this type of approach can be effective in influencing food practice (Kennedy et al., 1999).

The government White Paper, *Choosing Health* (DH, 2004b), supports the use of community action for tackling nutrition-related health inequalities at community level and the use of community health workers in delivery to facilitate the prevention process through health education and health promotion. As community food initiatives (CFIs) are becoming more widely used to tackle health inequalities, there is a need to demonstrate their effectiveness through evaluation.

CASE STUDY

The Community Cooks Scheme is a community-based intervention delivered in Knowsley, Liverpool. It aims to improve the diet of local people through increasing nutritional education and improving food-related skills, such as cooking and shopping, by utilising individuals indigenous to the local community to deliver a range of activities within the community including 'Cook and Eat' sessions and promotional events. The University of Chester was commissioned to evaluate the project to assess the effectiveness of the scheme in raising awareness of what constitutes a healthy diet and achieving a resultant diet-related behavioural change amongst participants in Knowsley. To examine the role of the Community Cook in facilitating these changes.

A multi-method approach incorporating structured questionnaires, interviews, focus groups and observations with participants and trainers (community cooks) enabled examination of a range of activities undertaken in relation to project objectives to assess impact at both an awareness raising and behavioural change level. Sampling was defined geographically, consisting of participants and employees of the Community Cooks scheme in Knowsley. Cohorts were purposely recruited for follow-up via semi-structured focus group interviews.

The scheme has changed the diet-related behaviour of participants. There was an increased awareness of what constitutes a healthy diet and healthy cooking practices across all participants from the most deprived wards of Knowsley as a result of participation in the scheme. Findings showed change or intention to change in terms of improving the healthiness of the diet, specifically for salt intake and fruit and vegetable intake. Findings demonstrate the importance of the peer educator role of the community cooks in addressing common barriers to change such as cooking skills, access and confidence in addition to knowledge of a healthy diet. Qualitative data supported these findings. The evaluation has demonstrated diet-related changes as a direct result of the Community Cooks' intervention and hence the importance of their role in facilitating change or intention to change.

CONCLUSION

Nutritional inequalities ensue from a combination of barriers and enablers relating to the patterns that shape the food culture of a community. Therefore addressing nutritional inequalities requires a multi-faceted approach utilising both structural changes (i.e. creating an environment conducive to change), and individual-level behaviour changes (selecting healthier food choices facilitated by enhanced self-efficacy due to greater comprehension of the association between diet and health and improved food-related skills). Community-based food initiatives are a method of transferring skills and direct health promotion efforts to lower socio-economic populations and achieve change in the short, medium and long term.

FURTHER READING

WHO (2004) *Guiding Principles for Feeding Infants and Young Children during Emergencies*. Geneva: WHO.

40 Commissioning and Public Health

Frances Wilson and Moyra Baldwin

DEFINITION

The chapter will consider commissioning in the context of promoting public health and wellbeing where the focus is to keep people healthy and independent not just to treat them when they are ill (DH, 2007a). Commissioning takes place at individual, local and strategic levels and demands partnership working between key organisations including the Primary Care Trusts (PCTs), practice-based commissioners (PBCs), local authorities and third-sector providers. Commissioning is essential to the future organisation and delivery of appropriate and effective health and social care services for individuals, communities and populations. It is the means by which providers of care can secure and offer the 'best value' (DH, 2006a, 2007b; Primary Care Group London Network for Nurses and Midwives, 2007) for local citizens, patients and taxpayers.

Commissioning has developed a specific language. According to Woodin (2006) different terminology used in different contexts, academic and policy documents has evolved and caused confusion. All definitions identify commissioning as a proactive and strategic function of local authorities and Primary Care Trusts, acting on behalf of the public. Commissioning involves planning, designing and implementing the range of services to meet a population's healthcare needs fairly, efficiently and effectively and includes prevention and early intervention. A glossary of common terms associated with commissioning is to be found in Box 40.1.

Box 40.1 *Commissioning and associated terms*

Commissioning healthcare definition:
'Commissioning is a strategic and proactive process of identifying the healthcare needs of a given population and prioritising services to meet the needs within the resources available. Commissioning embraces patient choice and voice' (DH, 2006b; Wade et al., 2006).

Social services definition:
'Commissioning is the process of specifying, securing and monitoring services to meet individuals' needs at strategic level. This applies to all services, whether they are provided by the local authority or by the private or voluntary sectors' (Social Services Inspectorate and Audit Commission website)

Practice-based commissioning:
involves practices receiving an indicative budget from their PCT from which they commission the most appropriate services for their patients.

Procurement:
the process of identifying a supplier within an environment of open competition to deliver best value. Procurement may involve competitive tendering, competitive quotation, single sourcing as well as stimulating the market through awareness raising and education.

(Continued)

The following key points focus on public health commissioning as an
activity and as a process.

KEY POINTS

- Commissioning is integral to contemporary public health and social
  care undertaken at different levels in organisations.
- The socio-political climate along with stakeholders influence the
  focus and impact of commissioning.
- Commissioning is a cycle of interrelated activities with the service
  user at the centre.
- Improvement in public health and wellbeing are the motivators for
  and the desired outcomes of commissioning.

DISCUSSION

The focus of commissioning at any level should be on the service users
and their carers but improvement in public health is determined not
merely by short-term health gain. Commissioning for public health
requires investment to secure sustained health improvement such as
lifestyle changes and behaviour that will have a positive long-term impact
on health and wellbeing, e.g. smoking cessation which has the potential to
lead to long-term benefits as well as immediate positive effects.

Following the banning of smoking in public places there is already
evidence of fewer hospital admissions relating to heart disease in

Scotland. (www.guardian.co.uk). Although this is the result of legislation, commissioners can use such evidence to inform future commissioning decisions.

Whilst commissioning is a strategic activity, the process emphasises the importance of partnership working between communities and commissioners (DH, 2007a). Terminology differs between the commissioning agencies but strong emphasis is placed on the centrality of the service user in commissioning by social services. In health services there is a strategic emphasis on the process; however, at practice-based commissioning level the focus is on consultation, greater choice and direct involvement in the design of individual patient-centred care packages (DH, 2007a). In delivering their commissioning responsibilities, PCTs and practice-based commissioners, working with local authorities and others, have two roles: as advocates for patients, and custodians of tax-payers' money (DH, 2005a).

Commissioning is integral to contemporary public health and social care services. Government policies encapsulate structured efforts of a society to improve individuals' health and wellbeing. Continuing with reforms the government in *Our Health, Our Care, Our Say* (DH, 2006e) set out its vision for improving the nation's health. Tackling health problems early, emphasis on prevention, early intervention and health promotion are essential to meet the needs of the population in the twenty-first century. Commissioning is essential to promoting public health.

The socio-political climate and stakeholders influence the focus and impact of commissioning. Using resources effectively has become increasingly important since the early years of the NHS. The concept of the 'internal market', originally advanced by Enthoven in 1985, along with a policy of achieving greater efficiency, is intended to re-establish the financial balance of the NHS and enable better care that is closer to home for patients. Committed to the public health agenda the Department of Health has driven the commissioning process, producing a plethora of policy and guidance documents. Making the NHS fit for the twenty-first century a 10-year programme of investment for reform began with the NHS Plan (DH, 2000b). Recent reconfiguration of strategic health authorities and PCTs, completed in 2007 and 2008 respectively, is the backdrop for commissioning today.

Commissioning is a cycle of interrelated activities at the centre of which is the individual/service user. The literature abounds with diagrammatic representations of commissioning as a cycle. Here we have synthesised these into the Commissioning Framework (Figure 40.1).

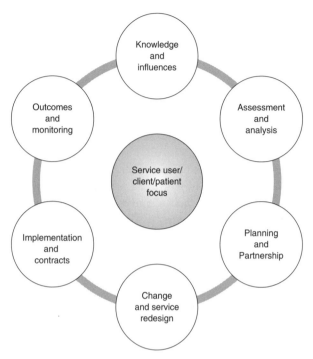

Figure 40.1 *The politico-economic climate of health and social care*

Knowledge and influences

To provide quality health and social care for a population, commissioners need a repertoire of relevant skills, knowledge and experience. Recent publications promote the development of competencies for world class commissioning (DH, 2007b) to support PCT activities. According to the Department of Health (2007a), skills for commissioning are underdeveloped. We would suggest that potential commissioners have existing and transferable skills which they need to identify and integrate into a flexible framework. To optimise the commissioning of sensitive and appropriate services commissioners require adequate support. Success depends on commissioning organisations recognising the educational requirements of the role. The subsequent implication is that education providers will supply opportunities for this development.

Assessment and analysis

Needs assessment is a systematic method of determining public health. It requires a robust evidence-based process involving analysis of data from a variety of sources including epidemiological studies, user surveys, stakeholder opinions, government directives as well as research-based interventions (DH, 2005c; NICE, 2005a).

Planning and partnership

Planning and collaborative partnership working are essential. A review of current provision, gap analysis, prioritisation and appraising the market capacity, including specifying the services and standard, are required (Woodin, 2006). The attributes required for 'world class commissioning' (DH, 2007b) are visionary and inspiring leadership, which we suggest is essential to enable modelling of future service requirements.

Change and service redesign

From the above, the decision commissioners are frequently faced with is service redesign. Such changes can have a significant impact on the workforce as roles may need to be revised or revoked. These may be viewed as either a positive or negative aspect of commissioning.

Implementation and contracts

Contracts are clearly set out agreements between the provider and commissioner. They state the objectives which will meet a population's specific health and social care needs. They set out the service specification and the quality standards to be achieved. Designing some service specifications is challenging because the services are poorly understood (http://www.rcslt.org/resources/managers_resources/service_spec).

Outcomes and monitoring

The types of contract and service specifications will have an impact on the monitoring processes as well as on the workforce. Outcomes need to reflect the aspirations of commissioning and be capable of measuring the short- and long-term health gain of the population, including the expected change in health status.

School nurses have the potential to improve outcomes for young people of school age by redefining the service they provide. Services need to be creatively shaped and changed not only to empower young people to make informed decisions but to promote choice, provide confidential advice and support, improve access, refer and signpost to other services and complement personal, social and health education programmes. The challenge is to ensure that services are delivered in the right place, at the right time by the right professional in a way that meets young people's needs. The commissioning process acts as an effective framework for school nurses to develop a clear vision of the future and provides a transparent strategy that places young people at the centre so that change happens effectively and efficiently.

Successful commissioning must be based on the common core values of the integration agenda. This will lead school nurses to review and map the services they currently offer young people and consider them against a broad needs analysis to provide a baseline for future provision. Services should consider all children of school age, including those who are vulnerable and the 'hard to reach' groups who may not always attend school.

Young people are key drivers of change and their views and participation must be integral to the change process if outcomes are to be achieved. Whilst the process will be driven by targets it should also be driven by quality, clinicians and potential health gain. Clear vision and leadership will therefore identify priorities and resources to plan and deliver a redesigned service in partnership with other agencies, to meet the needs of young people that can be measured year on year against agreed outcomes.

CONCLUSION

Improvement in public health and wellbeing are the motivators for and the desired outcomes of commissioning. It follows that commissioning is an organised and highly regulated activity in all aspects of its provision.

FURTHER READING

Department of Health (2007) *Commissioning Framework for Health and Wellbeing.* London: DH.

Wade, E., Smith, J., Peck, E. and Freeman, T. (2006) *Commissioning in the Reformed NHS: Policy into Practice.* Birmingham: University of Birmingham, Health Services Management Centre NHS Alliance.

key concepts in public health

Part III
Populations and Public Health Practice

41 Public Health and Mental Health

David Coyle

DEFINITION

The concept of mental health within a public health context is both obvious and paradoxical. The connection is obvious because everybody experiences psychological distress within their lives at some point. Though not everybody will experience such traumas to a debilitating degree, some will. The process by which a person's mental health is mediated is inherently wider than a biological or psycho-pathogenic model. It must also be a social one, defined by functional relationships, distress to self and others and a perception within wider society of differentness and often dangerousness.

The concept is paradoxical as an individual with a mental health problem is seen as unwell, psycho-pathogenic or as requiring treatments, care and adaptation (Oliver, 1996). The individual will be required to change, to be less unwell and more functional. This paradox places mental health problems within the person, though as we shall see, mental health is a diverse and complex concept and the role public health has in creating, maintaining and defending good mental health is a pivotal one and the responsibility of many. Mental ill health affects around one in six individuals within the UK (Singleton et al., 2000).

KEY POINTS

- Mental health promotion.
- The stigma of mental disorder and dangerousness impacts on policy.
- Inclusion as a means to live full lives for individuals and communities.
- Working together: individuals, communities and policy.

DISCUSSION

It seems that different populations are more susceptible to mental ill health. Women are more likely to suffer from depression than men

(Pilgrim and Rogers, 2003). Afro-Caribbean men are more likely to have a diagnosis of psychosis than Caucasian men of similar ages and some studies suggest that migration impacts negatively on mental health (Fernando, 2003; SCMH, 2004). Age as a factor in mental disorder is widely recognised. Transitional related events such as adolescence, stressful life events and biological degenerative conditions such as dementia affect many individuals.

There appears to be an inverse correlation of mental health between individuals from more and less privileged backgrounds. Those with higher levels of income and affluence are less likely to experience psychological distress than their less well off counterparts (Pilgrim and Rogers, 2003). Certain occupational groups appear to experience higher levels of mental disorder than others: people such as doctors, nurses, teachers, farmers and ex-servicemen are more likely to experience stress-related disorders (Taylor et al., 2007).

Mental health problems are estimated to cost Britain around £24 billion a year (SCMH, 2007). Therefore the issue of promoting good mental health and effectively supporting those affected is one that, in one way or another, affects us all.

It is clear then that to approach mental health with its diverse and complex aetiologies through a single medical or treatment approach would deal with only part of the problem. Any work or intervention should be aimed at a public health level, a community level as well as at an individual one. This chapter will not discuss causative factors as such that may lead to mental health problems as there are many competing theories. The reader is directed to other works such as Bentall (2003), and for biological causations to Blows (2003), for fuller discussions.

If, as already discussed, we will all experience a degree of mental distress and one in four of us will experience depression, then we cannot avoid mental ill health altogether. We can however mitigate its impact by identifying factors that promote positive mental wellbeing and those that may make us more vulnerable to distress. Mental health promotion was identified as standard 1 in the National Standards Framework for Mental Health (DH, 1999). Although pivotal in mental health policy over the past nine years, health promotion still lacks sound financial investment to support the activities required (Taylor et al., 2007).

Good mental health has been defined by the government as 'The emotional and spiritual resilience which enables enjoyment of life, and the ability to survive pain, disappointment and sadness; and as a positive sense of wellbeing and an underlying belief in our own and others' dignity and worth' (DH, 2001b: 28).

Mental health promotion can be defined as the process by which an individual or community is assisted in achieving a positive sense of well-being. However, to focus on the individual's resilience as the key to psychological happiness ignores the role that wider social and cultural factors play. McDonald (2006) argues strongly that government initiatives focusing on personal or individual interventions do not restore people; they simply offset the time when they will become distressed again. In other words, simply fixing the person, but not their housing, employment, community, equality or opportunity, will result in an inevitable recurrence of disorder.

McDonald and O'Hara (1998) describe a 10-element map providing an analysis based on Albee and Ryan-Finn (1993) where factors relating to mental health and wellbeing are articulated across individual and societal divides. Factors affecting mental health promotion include emotional processing, self-management skills, self-esteem, environmental quality, social alienation, stress, emotional negligence, emotional abuse, environmental deprivation and social participation. An individual's deficit in one area may be mediated or offset by strengths in another. For instance, someone living in a poor environment with little social contact may also have good self-management skills with low stress and high self-esteem. Further, the interrelationship between the state and legislative/social policy framework can be explored within the concept of micro; (the individual), exo (the close network, family), meso (community) and macro (legislature/social policy). This is more generally known as the social ecological model (Bronfenbrenner, 1979).

Stress as a factor exacerbating mental ill health should also be seen in context of stress in families – the exo level; (see Zubin and Spring, 1977), the community environment such as levels of crime, and in relation to policies in employment that minimise stress in the workplace, such as family friendly working and access to counselling or support. Finally, there is the macro level context relating to government policies that support families, provide access to health and wellbeing services and direct resources to those identified as being at greatest need.

With this in mind, government policy since 1999 has attempted to focus on tackling the factors that promote wellbeing at individual levels – Gateway workers (DH, 2003c), support time and recovery workers (DH, 2003e), cognitive behavioural therapists (DH, 2008b) – as well as creating positive and sustaining communities (ODPM, 2005) community regeneration, and removing barriers that create inequity and discrimination at a legislative and policy level (Disability Discrimination Act 1996; Human Rights Act 1998; DH, 2001b).

At the heart of policy over the last 10 years has been the rhetoric of joined up approaches across government. The assertion is that without the combined effort of departments, at local, national and central levels, focusing on housing, education, health, criminal justice and the environment, we cannot develop healthy and enriched lives. In theory the idea of departments and agencies working collaboratively without regard for their own influence is hopeful, but possibly naïve.

Groups that are marginalised or constitute a low political priority may not fall within the reach of stated policy. Mental illness has a stigma associated to it, one that government policy has sought to redress (DH, 2001b; DH, 2008b).

Government policy may also be accused of being contradictory when considering factors impacting on mental health. The DH (1999) standard 1 challenges the stigma of mental illness, as does *Making it Happen* (DH, 2001b). The Mental Health Act (2007) creates compulsory treatment in the community and, more worryingly, detention of people with personality disorder without being subject to the criminal justice system.

A joined up approach and partnership between the government, communities and the individual is laudable, but increasing individualisation of problems, physical and mental, contradicts the former. One does not choose mental illness in the way one makes lifestyle choices that impact on physical wellness, and therefore models of health promotion addressing physical public health may not be 'necessarily appropriate' for mental illness.

Further analysis would suggest the theoretical precursor to policy has its origins in the ideas of social capital (Putnam, 1995, 2000; Field, 2008). Here the determinants of individual functioning focus on the reciprocal relationships and networks within a culture or society, creating a sense of civic wellbeing and connectedness. Or as Putnam states: 'social capital refers to connections among individuals – social networks and the norms of reciprocity and trustworthiness that arise from them' (2007: 5). It has also been described by as Cote and Healy (2001: 33) as 'networks together with shared norms, values and understandings that facilitate co-operation within and among groups'.

Within mental health belonging and being a part of a community may be part of recovery, though as Putnam (2007) suggests, the decline in reciprocal relationships in communities is worrying and makes key outcomes such as removing the stigma of mental health and promoting social inclusion (DH, 1999) more challenging. Social inclusion, a part of social capital, may however be promoted by increasing an individual's resilience, coping skills, modified cognitions (through cognitive behavioural therapy), and/or by examining social capital in their environments. By exploring a community's opportunity for engagement, mapping a community's available venues and associations, and identifying key individuals whose influence in a community could be beneficial, the potential to increase face to face encounters with their known benefits become manifold (Lunt and Coyle, 2007).

The concept of social capital is heavy on rhetoric and light on evidence. It could nevertheless be a basis for interventions or strategies to improve the mental wellbeing of individuals and communities. Whilst the tangible evidence for one factor above others leading to a person's mental distress is thin, the relationships between civic connectedness, networks, support, inclusion, spirituality and neighbourliness appear important in determining the likelihood or risk of mental distress and, by the same measure, an individual's ability to recover function following an episode of distress.

CASE STUDY

James had become increasingly isolated and excluded from everyday contacts as his mental health problems endured over ten years. Having left his school friends to attend university where he experienced his first episode of psychosis. He lost contact with the few friends he made at his short time at university when he moved back to live with his mother. Without employment or relationships which define life for so many people; James' world was increasingly defined by contact with professionals and other supporters, his community psychiatric nurse and support worker. By thinking in a public health construct it is possible to create means that could maximise possibilities within his life by identifying areas of development in social relationships and activities that are valued by the person and by the wider community. By identifying people in James's circle of support (Lunt and Coyle, 2007) it is possible to strengthen relationships. People close to James can identify opportunities that create social inclusion. The supporters in James's life will develop both the capacity and motivation in finding roles and relationships that will define his life in terms other than as mental health sufferer.

CONCLUSION

The current evidence for psychological therapies is reasonably strong, indicating their use in supporting individuals manage distressing experiences (Kendrick et al., 2006; Taylor et al., 2007). The government's commitment to creating 3,500 more cognitive therapists (DH, 2008) is encouraging. Combination approaches of talking therapies and psychopharmacological treatment will alleviate the symptoms of many. But what of the causes that in combination lead an individual to experience mental distress? A public health model, maximising the opportunities for the individual within their community (Mental Health Foundation, 2000), would help connect people with the myriad groups, associations and organisations who, in partnership, may create and sustain 'a positive sense of wellbeing and an underlying belief in our own and others' dignity and worth'. In other words, good mental health.

FURTHER READING

Cattan, M. (2006) *Mental Health Promotion. A Life Span Approach*. London: Open University Press.
Field, J. (2008) *Social Capital*, 2nd edn. London: Routledge.

42 Adherence to Treatment – A Person-centred Approach

Dianne Phipps and Sara Bell

DEFINITION

In the discussions below, the term 'treatment' refers to any advised course of action within a public health context. This could be prescribed medication, or a behavioural change such as increased exercise.

Discussion continues as to how to describe what we have called adherence. The most popular terms to date are *compliance, concordance* and *adherence*.

Compliance can mean that the person is carrying out the recommended treatment (Horne, 2006), suggesting individuals are passive recipients of healthcare treatment or advice, not active parties in improving/maintaining their own health and wellbeing. This may cause difficulties: someone seen as 'non-compliant' may also be considered difficult or uncooperative. The term 'compliance' can be seen as passive, without due regard for individuals and their thoughts, opinions or actions.

'Concordance' is a more person-centred term, as agreeing the treatment is a joint decision between adviser and individuals. Concordance is an attempt to address the imbalance of power often present in healthcare communications between adviser and advised (Bell et al., 2007).

In recent literature, 'adherence' – meaning carrying out and sticking to the advised treatment – is now used, with 'high' and 'low' adherence behaviours being acceptable descriptions as opposed to 'good' or 'bad' adherence (NCCSDO, 2005).

Adherence to treatment is difficult to quantify: many people have failed to adhere to prescribed treatment and/or health advice, with 30–50 per cent of people considered to be non-adherent to treatment (Morris and Schulz, 1992; cited in Vermeire et al., 2001). Various methods have been used to measure adherence (patient diaries, prescription audits); overestimation remains an issue, and there is a recognised need for a way of measuring non-adherence (NCCSDO, 2005). The discussion and investigation of adherence is important for the public health professional for reasons of cost to individuals' health, and to services should the prescribed/advised treatment not be adhered to (Metcalfe, 2005).

KEY POINTS

- Best practice/treatment/advice is only beneficial if recipients carry out the advice or take the treatment.
- Non-adherence does not lie solely with patients. Poor information given by advisers, badly written information leaflets, and communication breakdowns may be factors.
- Individuals' perception of adequate information may be different from the information giver's.
- Working in a person-centred way, for the public health practitioner, may be the best way to support individuals in adhering to their treatment/advice regime.

DISCUSSION

There are many reasons, both intentional and unintentional, why people do not adhere to their treatment regimens or advice. Possible reasons are:

- Suggested treatments may interfere so much with the person's everyday life that they think it not worth the known benefits to continue.
- Treatments may be complex and/or long term.
- Individuals may not have had, or not have understood, the information provided.
- It could be due to depression, stress and anxiety.
- Person may be forgetting to take prescribed medication.
- Deciding not to take prescribed medication: individuals may disagree with the treatment, or may decide not to take it e.g. because they feel better (or worse!)
- It could be due to mental health status.
- There may be communication issues between adviser and individuals.
- Individuals may not believe that the medication will do them good (Skinner, 2004; Myers and Midence, 1998).

Individuals may be affected by several of these reasons: for example diabetic children may need help to incorporate the treatment regime into their lifestyle or to remember to take medication, and may not fully understand all the reasons for the treatments. Indeed, adherence is greatest where people are most dependent on help and support (Morris and Schulz, 1992; cited in Vermeire et al., 2001) – the more support given, the better the chance of compliance, as with children whose wellbeing may be overseen by parents. Age is also positively correlated to adherence (Metcalfe, 2005). However, in some instances rebellion against treatment is a reaction to nagging family or friends: teenagers are often non-compliant, and are rebelling from a sense of indestructibility.

The reasons for non-adherence are very personal, and the adviser may never know the true reasons why their suggestions have been disregarded. Ferner (2003) states: 'We should hardly be surprised that our patients wish to hide their failings from us.' People dislike being chastised for forgetting medication, or admitting that they did not understand the explanations given or the leaflet provided.

Sometimes the reason for non-adherence does not lie solely with patients. Poor information given by advisers, badly written information leaflets, and communication breakdowns between the two parties could be influences. Richards, et al. (2005) suggest that a major factor is how satisfied patients feel with the consultation. The quality of listening and explanation, and the perception of the health practitioner's interpersonal skills, is significantly related to patient satisfaction and adherence.

How can adherence be improved? One suggestion for improving adherence to medication (researched specifically with older people) is a multi-method approach, the AIDES method (Bergman-Evans, 2006), which could be adapted to suit individual needs (Box 42.1).

Box 42.1

A Assessment: this could include assessment of individuals' capacity for understanding and retaining information, and memory function.

I Individualisation: adherence is more likely if the treatment/advice is tailored to the individuals' needs.

D Documentation: if appropriate to the individuals' needs, this helps communication between adviser and advised, providing a focus for discussion.

E Education: again, tailored specifically for the individuals.

S Supervision: coupled with evaluation of the regimen, so both parties can discuss what works best or is inconvenient.

Each of these items can be interpreted differently, which can increase or reduce adherence, e.g. education – individuals' perception of adequate information is possibly different from the information giver's (Ekman et al., 2007).

Working in a person-centred way, for the public health practitioner, may be the best way to encourage individuals to adhere to their treatment regime, as recommended by Aronson (2007): 'Tailor the treatment to the patient's lifestyle, not the other way round.'

The AIDES model clearly outlines the need for joint working between adviser and advised, and is person centred, but how practical is this approach for all aspects of public health work? The best approach may well be a multi-method approach encompassing Bergman-Evans' suggestions. Katz (1997) developed basic patient education guidelines for providers, which although 10 years older encompasses aspects of the AIDES method (Bergman-Evans, 2006). Katz' six steps are simplified as:

- Limit discussion to three or four points during each encounter.
- Use simple everyday language.
- Supplement oral instructions with written material.
- Involve the patient's family members or significant others.
- Ask the patient to restate recommendations to you.
- Repeat and reinforce the concepts that were discussed.

Methods such as these can be seen within some learning disability services, especially in such documentation as health needs assessments.

A number of theoretical models have been put forward to account for complex health-related behaviours. Kinzie (2005), Miller and Rollnick (2002) believe that health behaviour change involves three essential constructs:

- patients' readiness for change;
- perceived importance of change;
- one's ability to change (self-efficacy).

Interventions addressing these have proven effective in improving adherence among those with a wide range of illnesses (Rains et al., 2006).

The social learning theory of Bandura (1986) indicates that confidence in one's ability to perform an action (self-efficacy) and the expectation that behaviour will have a desirable result (outcome-efficacy) are important mediators of performance. Self-efficacy is a more powerful indicator of adherence. Rains et al. (2006) highlight that skills to carry out various health behaviours are not sufficient to ensure they are performed; rather, patients must believe they possess the skills and that these behaviours will achieve the desired outcomes.

CASE STUDY

Jeremy, a 23-year-old man living with his parents, was diagnosed as developmentally delayed when aged 4. He attended a local special school until age 19 when he started part time employment.

Jeremy's mother has referred him to the community learning disability nurse (CLDN) as she is concerned about excessive alcohol intake. The nurse visits Jeremy at home, and he agrees to have his parents present while the nurse carries out an assessment.

Jeremy tells the nurse that he goes out four times a week to the local pub, having approximately seven pints of lager and four double brandies on each occasion. Jeremy admits that sometimes he feels unwell the morning after, and sometimes has been late or missed work. His manager has asked to see him about this. Jeremy's mother confirms this, stating she has picked him up several times from his friend's house when he was unable to walk home. His mother is obviously concerned and often sits by his bed at night when he arrives back, in case he vomits.

The CLDN makes another appointment to visit. The case is discussed with the nurse's supervisor and a course of action agreed.

Upon returning, the nurse talks to Jeremy alongside his mother (Jeremy is still happy with this). The nurse produces materials with which to talk through appropriate drinking with Jeremy. Jeremy understands the health implications of his drinking, and agrees to cut down. Neither he nor his mother think they need further visits, nor want to be referred to other services.

A month later, Jeremy is re-referred, again due to his drinking. When the nurse rings to make an appointment, Jeremy answers and asks if he can see the nurse alone.

At the visit, the nurse discovers that Jeremy continues to drink as he goes to the pub with his work colleagues and girlfriend. Jeremy states that if he didn't drink, he couldn't go out and would not have any social life at all, nor girlfriend, whom his mother does not know about and who he doesn't feel he could bring back home.

CONCLUSION

The public health practitioner, knowing that adherence to treatment is a real issue in healthcare, needs to work with individuals in a person-centred way to ensure that best advice becomes best action on the part of the advised.

Practitioners must listen to individuals for important factors such as mistrust, fear and unrealistic doubts. These need to be addressed and resolved. Simple regimes, written information and effective practitioner–patient communication and partnership may be helpful in positively influencing adherence.

FURTHER READING

Mental Health Specialist Library (2008) *Hot topics – our most popular sections*. Retrieved 28 March 2008, from http://www.nelmh.org/page_view.asp?c=1&fc=001006&did=1502

Miller, W.R. and Rollnick, S. (2002) *Motivational Interviewing: Preparing People for Change*, 2nd edn. New York: Guildford.

Myers, L. B. and Midence, L. (1998) *Adherence to Treatment in Medical Conditions*. London: Harwood Academic.

43 Public Health and the Pre-school Child

Jean Mannix and John Horley

DEFINITION

Child public health (CPH) can be defined as 'the organised efforts of society to develop public health policies to promote children's and young people's health, to prevent disease in children and young people and to foster equity for children and young people, within a framework of sustainable development' (Kohler, 1998).

CPH should arguably be viewed as potentially the most important and effective public health activity in health and social care practice. The key aims are health promotion and protection and disease prevention. Practitioners working with children and families must focus on addressing the wider determinants of health with parents while contributing to meaningful CPH, thus improving the health and wellbeing of future populations. For this, practitioners must work collaboratively with parents, agencies and groups, to develop realistic aims for disease prevention and early intervention strategies to improve health.

KEY POINTS

- CPH involves detection, promotion and prevention strategies.
- Advocacy has a key function within CPH.
- CPH strategies require leadership.
- Collaborative partnership and inter-agency working are crucial to CPH activities.

DISCUSSION

The context of CPH is all-encompassing. The very essence of CPH needs to be deeply embedded and integrated into the practitioner's everyday working with families, children and communities, along with cognisance of wider socio-political issues such as housing, employment and education. The Acheson Report (1998) stated that health inequalities are associated with a number of social, socio-economic and individual factors, many of them more common in people living in deprived areas. Although establishing cause and effect is difficult, specific risk factors could be targeted and child health improved by reducing these inequalities. However, whilst individuals cannot control factors such as age, genetics and sex, individual lifestyle, particularly of parents, also plays a part in CPH.

Consequently, to improve children's health and wellbeing one must strip away layers of inter-generational influence, promote individual health and wellbeing, and invest in improving outcomes for children. Tackling the multi-factorial layers at different levels, from individuals to populations, is essential to make an impact upon the range of issues involved (Blair et al., 2004). Health promotion at an early stage should improve health and wellbeing for the adult population, at the same time being a cost-effective approach for future generations.

Essentially, public health is concerned with prevention, promotion and protection; however, this is difficult in CPH as children are under their parents' influence. Consequently, interventions must be targeted towards parents in order to realise benefits for future generations. The review of health visiting, *Facing the Future* (DH, 2007e), adopted the concept of progressive universalism, recommending investment in intensive home visiting for children and families. Home visiting is a key indicator for improved health outcomes for children and families, as quality of the home environment predicts children's cognitive and social development (Kitzman et al., 2000; Engelke and Engelke, 1992). Health visitors and midwives are ideally placed to develop early intervention strategies with families during home visits. Unfortunately, intensive home visiting is restricted to a very small number of very complex families. Health visitors currently undertake universal home visiting, and intensive home visiting must not replace it but remain an additional service. *The Child Health Promotion Programme* (CHPP) (DH, 2008), part of the *National Service Framework for Children, Young People and Maternity Services* (DH, 2004d), has clarified the role of progressive universalism, setting out an integrated approach to supporting children and families with the aim of improving the health and wellbeing of children (but clearly stating that health visitors will co-ordinate and lead the CHPP rather than deliver it in isolation).

As research demonstrates that home visiting is a key factor in CPH, it is essential that universal home visiting is maintained and agencies work together to develop effective CPH strategies. Kitzman et al. (2000) found health outcomes were improved greatly with families who had home visits rather than clinic attendance alone. The government's vision to align the Public Service Agreements (PSA) indicators to prevention and early intervention strategies and to measure outcomes ensures that CPH is a priority for local commissioners. The PSA indicators are intrinsically linked to the *Every Child Matters* (DfES, 2003) five outcomes:

- Be healthy.
- Stay safe.
- Enjoy and achieve.
- Make a positive contribution.
- Achieve economic wellbeing.

The government's current policy drivers (DH, 2004a, 2004b, 2007e; DCSF, 2007; DH, 2008) intend that every child, whatever their background or circumstances, should have the support needed to achieve these outcomes. Understanding of health inequalities is crucial for policy development and early interventions to support CPH, including directing services depending on health needs assessment. Conversely, achieving these outcomes requires uniting statutory and voluntary organisations providing services for children and families, encouraging innovation and new ways of working together. Collaboration – sharing information and working together to promote CPH and identify services in a non-stigmatising way (DH, 2008) – is essential, thereby engaging with children and families to develop meaningful partnerships to assist in the delivery of early interventions.

CPH is complex due to multi-factorial and inter-generational elements which have a direct impact upon health, consequently requiring sustained investment and commitment from commissioners of services, the government and the key agencies involved – namely health, education and social care – to ensure co-ordinated approaches. This does not necessarily mean that these agencies have to deliver the required children and family services.

Ultimately, long-term investment in CPH requires measurable outcomes for children and families. Due to lack of measurable outcomes and evidence, earlier CPH was often inadequately resourced and under-researched. The *Children's Plan* (DCSF, 2007) has ambitious targets for 2020, linked intrinsically to the *Every Child Matters* five outcomes. Parents' and children's needs are highlighted in both the *Children's Plan* and the CHPP (DH, 2008), which state that future investment in integrated services will put children's and families' needs at the centre of service delivery. Policy drivers for CPH have now been developed, and it is currently implementation and evaluation which are crucial for the future public health of children and young people. As the *Children's Plan* states, leadership and collaboration are required to develop a 'world class workforce able to provide highly personalised support, so we will continue to drive up quality and capacity of those working in the children's workforce' (DCSF, 2007: 83).

It is essential that children and young people have a say in the public health issues affecting them as individuals and collectively. Children under 5 are often an invisible population lacking the freedom to make choices and influenced by others, especially parents, grandparents and the media. A fundamental need for CPH practitioners is to engage and support parents, as children's health remains dependent upon parents'. Leadership and advocacy are the key to engagement with parents, particularly with hard to reach families. By working in partnership with, and using strategies such as facilitation and empowerment, parents may be encouraged to set their own health goals and take responsibility for their own and their children's health. This is complex and dependent upon factors such as time, resource availability, commitment, mutual respect and, perhaps more importantly, trust between all parties. However, to promote the future health of populations, CPH must be given meaningful consideration by all who have a responsibility to improve child health. Finding strategies to protect and promote the health and wellbeing of children is essential. Though inter-professional and cross-agency working is challenging, solutions need to be developed and sustained in order to achieve the five *Every Child Matters* (DfES, 2003) outcomes and, more importantly, ensure a healthy future for children.

CASE STUDY

Jessica is a young mother of three children under 5 living in a small house in a deprived area. Jessica has been in care for short periods of time throughout her adolescence, mainly due to domestic abuse and her mother's mental health. Jessica has become increasingly concerned and aware of her weight gain. She has tried to lose weight in the past, but has gained weight with each pregnancy and is now four stone overweight. Jessica's diet is high in saturated fat with very little vegetables or fruit. All three children are in the 75th centile for weight and 25th centile for height. All children regularly attend the local children's centre with Jessica, and the staff undertake cookery sessions and encourage children to eat different types of food, especially fruit and vegetables. When the youngest was born, Jessica was diagnosed with post-natal depression; lethargy and the prescribed medication have further impacted on her weight gain.

Sally, the health visitor, has noticed a positive change in Jessica since the family have been attending the children's centre. Jessica's confidence and ability to cope with the children has improved slowly and she also breast-fed the youngest until he was 6 months old. Unfortunately Jessica's lifestyle choices impact upon her and the children, which frequently results in her failing to consider the children's and her own needs.

Sally has suggested lifestyle changes occasionally, but without success. Jessica has recently become friendly with another young mother who has stopped smoking and started to try to lose weight and eat more healthily; this has influenced Jessica to consider changing her own lifestyle.

Jessica asked Sally at a home visit for support to lose weight and about activities for families. Sally was able to work with Jessica on an individualised action plan that incorporated Jessica's own specific goals for weight loss and improved diet. Sally was able to advise Jessica of two local school/community initiatives – a 'five a day' campaign and a 'walking for health' initiative for children and families – which have been developed in partnership with education, social services, the local council, PCT and service users as part of the local obesity strategy.

CONCLUSION

This chapter has explored the concept of CPH from a number of perspectives. We have found that the ever changing arena of CPH requires partnership working with parents and agencies, and joint planning and commissioning of integrated services with other agencies, service users and, more importantly, parents. There is a shift in children and family services with new policy directives, redesign of services and the requirement to measure outcomes in relation to PSA indicators. It is essential that practitioners are attentive to children's and parents' needs while focusing on the CPH agenda and the inequalities that exist.

FURTHER READING

Blair, M., Stewart-Brown, S., Waterson, T. and Crowther, R. (2004) *Child Public Health*. Oxford: Oxford University Press.

Hall, D. and Elliman, D. (2006) *Health for All Children*. Oxford: Oxford University Press.

44 Public Health and the Schools Community

Gabrielle Rabie

DEFINITION

The school has been identified as a key 'setting' for the health and education of children and young people (DH, 2005d). Healthy settings are defined as 'the place or social context in which people engage in daily activities in which environmental, organizational, and personal factors interact to affect health and wellbeing' (WHO, 1998).

The National Healthy School Programme (NHSP) is a national standards framework (DfES, 1999), (predecessor to Department for Children, Schools and Families: DCSF) guiding the work of local partnerships between Primary Care Trusts (PCTs) and local education authorities (LEAs) in promoting a whole school approach to addressing specific health themes within schools. The programme is jointly sponsored by the Department of Health and the DCSF and managed by the Health Development Agency (HDA). The partnerships receive national funding and deliver on national targets set by the Department of Health (DH) and the DCSF (DH, 2004d).

KEY POINTS

- In the context of public health, the NHSP is based on a reciprocal relationship between education and health.
- Educational attainment plays a key role in determining health status and in breaking the cycle of health inequalities, and healthier children perform better academically.

NHSP:

- makes a specific contribution to health improvement and achieving health inequality targets, by promoting social inclusion and raising pupil achievement;
- has a key contribution to make to local preventive strategies for children, community and neighbourhood renewal strategies;
- contributes to national priorities.

DISCUSSION

The concept of 'healthy settings' as a resource for improving the health and wellbeing of populations originated from the World Health Organization (WHO) strategy, *Targets for Health for All* (1985) and was later refined by the Ottawa Charter for Health Promotion (1986), the Sundsvall Statement of 1992 and the Jakarta Declaration of 1997; cited by Wenzal (1997). According to Wenzal (1997) the term 'setting' is not a fundamental or strategic characteristic of health promotion but a tactical label representing the direction of measures to be taken by health professionals to improve the health status of selected population groups.

Schools offer a unique setting in which to target the health and well-being of children and young people. Recognition that pupils in a poor state of health will suffer from delayed learning and lower academic attainment has been reported by Devaney et al. (1993), the World Bank (1993). However, schools as a public health setting were first recognised in 1892 with the appointment of the first school nurse to look after the health of children in Chancery Lane school. The subsequent development of the school medical service mirrored the development of the education system in the early twentieth century and in 1904 Interdepartmental Committee on Physical Deterioration made forceful recommendations on how to improve child health which included training for mothers, the need for health societies, feeding arrangements for schoolchildren and combating juvenile smoking etc.

The National Healthy School Standard (NHSS) – introduced in 1999 and relaunched in 2005 as the NHSP – has its foundation in partnership and collaborative working between health and education. Based on a whole school approach it has four key themed areas: personal, social and health education (including sex and relationship education and drugs education), healthy eating, physical activity, and emotional health and wellbeing (EHWB) (including anti-bullying policy and practice). Attainment of 'healthy school' status is dependent on achievement of the national quality NHSP standards. Currently 94 per cent of schools are participating (20,815 schools) and 53 per cent of schools have national healthy school status (11,646 schools): that translates to about 3.7 million children and young people currently enjoying the benefits of a healthy school (DfES, 2007b).

The evidence base (although still in its infancy) demonstrates a positive impact. Schools involved in the NHSP report improvements in the management and support of pupils and have higher scores related to social inclusion indicators at Ofsted inspection (Ofsted, 2001; Aggleton et al., 2004, in DH, 2004d). Outcomes for pupils from deprived backgrounds educated in a 'healthy school' are improving in terms of behaviour, and standards of work (Ofsted, 2001), while Aggleton et al. (2004), in a qualitative comparison of secondary schools engaged in the NHSP with other secondary schools, reported that students in the NHSP schools were less likely to use illegal substances, were more likely to know where to access free condoms, were more at ease with the doctor and demonstrated higher levels of self-esteem. Fear of bullying in primary schools was also reported to be lower in the NHSP school (Aggleton et al., 2004). However the Health Development Agency (DH, 2004d) suggests that proving causality between school-based interventions and improved health and achievement in the student population is fraught with difficulties as school are complex environments where multiple influences on health are impossible to control for.

The NHSP *Final Evaluation Report* (2004) concludes that participation in the NHSS improved the status of health-related work in schools, and worked best where partners had a history of working together and a shared understanding of improving health in schools. NHSS has provided a useful infrastructure through which health-related work can take place with schools. However there was little quantitative data to demonstrate differences between schools at Level 3 (highest level) of the NHSS and other schools. This lack of data was related to the 'localness and the individualness' of projects within the NHSP and the difficulty of extrapolation of the local data to national levels. DeBell (2007: 106) argues that the NHSP from its outset was a teacher-led initiative and that this may have slowed initial health progress due to absence of health sector representation in many of the key decision-making bodies that led the NHSP in the early years.

CASE STUDY

The media has placed much emphasis on binge drinking and young people. As a specialist community public health nurse (SCPHN) you know that a number of young people in the school have been admitted to the local Accident and Emergency department for treatment. You are working with the individuals but are concerned that this is too little, too late and would like to target health promotion at the younger age groups before 'drinking' becomes an issue. Confidentiality must be maintained.

Practical application of the concept

The NHSP provides a framework for the inclusion of health-enhancing activities within the school setting. The evidence suggests that a whole school approach is the most effective model for the delivery of the NHSS. 'Binge drinking' could be suggested to the Healthy Schools council as an area for concern and a possible topic for the school to discuss. Utilising a whole school approach, the topic of alcohol and its effects could be introduced into the school curriculum for the target group.

The school council could undertake a pupil survey about what would enable them to resist the pressure to become involved in binge drinking.

Chemistry and Biology lessons might explore the short-, medium- and longer-term consequences of binge drinking on health and wellbeing, the Maths department could look at the cost of alcohol in relation to health and justice. Humanities might debate the history of alcohol and whether it would be licensed in light of current knowledge. The Physical Education department might explore the effects of alcohol on competitive performance. Personal, Social, Health and Citizenship Education and Sociology might explore the social and legal consequences of binge drinking. A 'peer' education scenario (which could be presented at school assemblies and parents evenings) could be developed in conjunction with the Drama department.

Parents could be engaged to support the programme by the provision of information sessions and leaflets to increase their own knowledge about alcohol and its effects. The local PCT could support the programme by providing specialist expert input regarding health-related issues and perhaps by jointly funding some of the human and material resources required to establish such a programme.

The involvement of the local authority Youth Services, ConneXions, emergency services and the voluntary sector in the school would facilitate dissemination of the key messages into the wider community, enabling the engagement of owners of licensed premises.

Evaluation of the process and outcomes of the programme and dissemination of the lessons learned would be essential to promote and replicate excellent practice.

CONCLUSION

Evidence suggests that young children who adopt unhealthy behaviours are more likely than others to continue these habits into adulthood (Barton and Parry-Jones, 2004), that educational attainment plays a key role in determining future health status and that healthy children perform better academically (DH, 2004b; DfES, 2003). Partnership and collaboration are the driving tenets of public health; since 1999 the government has made funding available to local education and health partnerships to support the development of the NHSP. Evaluation of the NHSP has demonstrated a positive impact, particularly in relation to the some of the key Ofsted indicators such as behaviour and inclusion. The evidence for positive health-related outcomes is less clear but as these outcomes are longer term it is difficult to judge. Health professionals need to become more fully engaged with the NHSP at all levels.

The NHSS provides a framework for the delivery of health promotion messages and activities within the school setting.

FURTHER READING

DeBell, D. (ed.) (2007) *Public Health Practice and the School Age Population*. London: Hodder Arnold.

Department for Education and Skills (1999) *National Healthy Schools Standard Guidance*. Retrieved 20 January 2008, from www.wiredforheath.gov.uk/PDF/ Brochurenew.pdf

Department of Health (2005) *National Healthy Schools Status: a guide for schools*. Retrieved 20 January 2008, from http://www.wiredforhealth.gov.uk/PDF/NHSS_ A_Guide_for_Schools_10_05.pdf

Health Development Agency (2004) *National Healthy Schools Programme: a briefing for directors of public health*. Retrieved 20 January 2008, from www.wiredforhealth. gov.uk/PDF/directors_briefing_04.pdf

45 Public Health and Young People

Gabrielle Rabie and Irene Cooke

DEFINITION

When considering the definition of 'young people', one needs to take into account the context of youth within society. According to Firth (2005) youth is a sociological category rather than a biological one. However, the World Health Organization (WHO, 1993) primarily uses a biological approach when it defines 'young people' as being between the ages of 10 and 24 years, and the term 'adolescence' as applying to the years from 10 to 19, with 'youth' determined as within the age range of 15 and 24 years. The WHO (2004) however recognises the limitations of using chronological definitions as they often fail to reflect the biological, psychological and social factors that influence the period of transition from child to adult. Thus the definition is contested, with a range of opinions being offered.

In terms of demography, it is reported that adolescents account for 13–15 per cent of the total population of the United Kingdom, and it is predicted that this figure will have grown by a further 8.5 per cent between 1998 and 2011. Young people are therefore a considerable resource for the future health of the nation. Mortality rates for those under the age of 15 years continue to fall, with the leading cause of death in this age group being accidents, followed by cancer (ONS, 2003; Barton and Parry-Jones, 2004). However, a significant number of adolescents are now living with increased morbidity, which is mainly due to a chronic condition being diagnosed during childhood (DfES, 2005).

KEY POINTS

- All young people experience transition during their lives.
- A number of young people live with a long-term medical condition.

DISCUSSION

The study of public health policy and young people has sought to address some of the problems associated with youth, such as teenage pregnancy, sexually transmitted diseases, alcohol, cigarette and illegal substance misuse, mental health, obesity, low educational achievement, crime, disorder and unemployment (DH, 2004d). It is argued that this exhaustive list over-represents 'problems' associated with youth, and primarily ignores the majority of young people who make a successful and healthy transition from childhood to adulthood despite the influence of the media, sedentary lifestyle, promiscuity and the availability of cigarettes alcohol and drugs (Barton and Parry-Jones, 2004).

Today's young people have not had the benefit of accessing early intervention and Sure Start programmes as children, and consequently are unable to 'catch up' as they journey along the continuum from dependent child to independent adult. Lifestyle behaviour is fundamentally important throughout the adolescent years, as there is a strong likelihood that lifestyle choices which are made during adolescence will be continued into adulthood (Barton and Parry-Jones, 2004). It is therefore vitally important that young people are aware of the potential benefits and threats to their health when making lifestyle choices, and that public health policy and strategies comprehensively embrace these themes to empower individuals.

Transition

Definitions of transition differ, but most agree that transition involves a passage of change (Kralik et al., 2006). Bridges (2004: xii) encapsulated the concept as being 'not an event, but rather the "inner reorientation and self-redefinition" that people go through in order to incorporate change into their life'. It appears to be a continuous process in which the young person is dependent upon self-awareness and insight in order to make the change.

The young adult experiences greater and more frequent changes than at almost any other period in their life: these include passing the biological milestone of puberty (Bynner, 2005), and psychological and emotional changes (Barton and Parry-Jones, 2004).

There are a number of key identifiable transitions which the young person experiences within education, such as the hierarchical nature of the transition from being a senior in the primary school to becoming one of the newest students in the secondary school. This may pose challenges related to self-esteem. Also, the move from high school to college or university can result in friendship and location alterations (HM Treasury, 2004; DfES, 2007b). Social transitions feature during this time, for example leaving home and finding employment or becoming unemployed. Economic viability may subsequently be experienced for the first time. Teenage parenthood features for a number of young people (DH, 2004d). Given that the transition is dependent upon the young person having insight and self-awareness, the process of change may prove challenging.

An interesting point is made by Barton and Parry-Jones (2004) who report that the individual undergoes two developmental transitions during their life; the first phase being from childhood to adolescence, and the second phase being the transition from adolescence to adulthood, which, they argue, is being increasingly protracted. It appears that the continuum from dependence to independence is extending, and one explanation given is the prolongation of adult education which may affect economic independence.

The changing social environment in which young individuals live may affect their contact with significant others, such as parents and friends, and present new challenges as they navigate through life without access to the familiar support systems they have previously relied on (HM Treasury, 2004; DfES, 2007b).

It is evident that young people undergo the challenges of transition on numerous occasions during their life; however, the majority are usually able to deal successfully with issues over a period of time (Coleman and Hendry, 1999) and make the transition to adult life without experiencing serious or lasting difficulties (DfES, 2005). Nevertheless, for some young people the transition can be problematic. This is particularly evident for those individuals who do not have stable networks at home, for example as the homeless or those who are in care (DfES, 2005).

Disabled young people experience another type of transition which primarily relates to the transition from a child-focused to an adult-oriented healthcare system (DH, 2006f). This may affect those who have a chronic physical or mental health condition from childhood. The individuals' needs should be comprehensively and sensitively addressed in these cases so the transition experienced is continuous and seamless.

Long-term conditions

Long-term conditions such as diabetes, asthma, epilepsy, cystic fibrosis and sickle cell disease can have a major impact on young people's lives (DH, 2007a) and may be either continued from childhood or experienced for the first time in adolescence (Barton and Parry-Jones, 2004).

Currently 5–10 per cent of adolescents live with a long-term conditions or disability; however, these figures are projected to rise given the advancements in research and medical technology whereby young people are now surviving conditions which would previously have been fatal (DH, 2006f; Barton and Parry-Jones, 2004). It is estimated that almost one in five children can be expected to be a heavy user of health services by virtue of having a chronic long-term condition or disability (Woodroffe et al., 1993).

The aim of care for young people should be to provide the majority of their treatment within the community so that they can lead as normal a life as possible (DH, 2007b). This has recently been reinforced by 'You're Welcome Quality Criteria' (DH, 2007b), which identifies that all young people are entitled to receive appropriate healthcare. An adolescent takes increasing responsibility for their own health as they develop throughout the teenage years (Barton and Parry-Jones, 2004), and therefore they need to be recognised as active partners in decisions regarding their health, which will empower them to embrace these new responsibilities. Collaboration with other agencies and services, such as schools, is essential for this to occur and to enable young people to make informed choices relating to their health. It is also recognised that taking risks, experimenting and pushing boundaries is an important part of growing up (DH, 2004c; DSCF, 2007b). Some individuals may choose to ignore their medical condition, which is termed 'adaptive denial' (Barton and Parry-Jones, 2004). In these cases, a partnership and concordant approach which is cognisant of the individuals' social interpretation of their health is essential in establishing the underlying rationale in respect of health and lifestyle choices.

CASE STUDY

Jack is a 13-year-old in year 8 of his secondary school. He lives with his parents and 11-year-old sister. Jack was diagnosed with asthma three years ago, and has begun to manage his condition independently. However, he has been admitted to hospital three times in the last 12 months due to acute exacerbations of his asthma. During discussions, it appears that Jack has not been taking the medication to manage his asthma as prescribed, because of feeling embarrassed about using his inhalers in front of his school friends. This also is making Jack 'feel different' and marginalised from the others in his class.

As a result of this, the school nurse organised a meeting between Jack and his parents, Jack's general practitioner, and the asthma specialist nurse to discuss how best to support Jack in taking his prescribed medication to prevent further acute exacerbation of his condition. It was decided that Asthma Awareness sessions could be introduced within the school, with input from the Drama department in respect of breathing exercises. Jack and his school friends would be invited to attend along with other interested students in order to raise awareness of asthma. The Physical Education department decided to ban aerosol deodorants and sprays to reduce the likelihood of initiating asthma attacks in pupils.

At the end of the Asthma Awareness sessions, Jack and his friends, and others who had attended, were awarded a Certificate of Attendance, and Jack was able to manage his condition independently and without requiring further hospital admissions.

CONCLUSION

Concerns are expressed regarding almost every aspect of the lifestyle behaviour of young people and its consequential impact on the health of the future nation. Patterns of behaviour are often set early in life (HM

Treasury, 2004; DfES, 2007b), and the young adult is at one of the critical stages of development regarding health-related behaviours (DH, 2004b). In seeking to address the public health concerns relating to young people we have briefly explored opportunities for effective direct interventions which both value and empower the young person as an individual with a right to self-determination. It can be argued that young people are not a homogeneous group and due consideration should be given to their diverse characteristics, which public health policy should seek to reflect.

There is a need to comprehensively address the critical points in young people's lives from a public health perspective as they are the future population of the nation, and our future – as well as theirs – depends on it.

FURTHER READING

Breinbauer, C. and Maddaleno, M. (2005) *Youth Choices and Change: Promoting Healthy Behaviours in Adolescents.* Washington: World Health Organization.

Coleman, J.C. (2007) *Adolescence and Health.* London: Wiley.

DeBell, D. (ed.) (2007) *Public Health Practice and the School Age Population.* London: Hodder Arnold.

McDougall, T. (ed.) (2006) *Child and Adolescent Mental Health Nursing.* Oxford: Blackwell.

46 Public Health and Adults

Sue Phillips

DEFINITION

Public health is a contested and contradictory term given the wide range of competing perspectives, priorities and services that it claims to deliver (Laverack, 2005). It is perhaps not surprising that many health and social care professionals, and others such as town planners, transport directors and voluntary agencies, would not see themselves as being involved in 'public health'. It is likely that public opinion would also see public health as being 'someone else's remit', and might consider its concerns to be drains or sanitation, or infectious diseases. However, public health, although it perhaps still belongs primarily to people employed in the health sector, in practice should belong to everyone. Earle suggests that public health consists of:

> a range of activities, performed by different people in a variety of settings and levels, and is thus both complex and diverse. It includes people working within different paradigms, or worldviews and ... with different yet over-lapping sets of values. (Earle, 2007: 7)

Hunter (2003: 36) argues that a better term is 'the health of the public' and 'the quality of life lived, rather than the absence of disease'. To this extent, it is the responsibility of every adult.

KEY POINTS

- Public health concerns everyone, on personal and professional levels.
- Should people be responsible for their own health? To what extent does this responsibility extend to the health of others?
- Individual versus collective responsibility; the role of legislation in controlling health behaviour.

DISCUSSION

Whose responsibility?

It is worrying when some healthcare professionals deem 'public health work' to be a specified activity, usually involving a relatively short time span, carried out by professionals who have 'public health' specifically included in their job title or description. In this way they dissociate themselves from having anything to do with it. According to Kelly and Symonds (2003: 127), nurses, for example, have been led into a blind alley where they are more responsible for interventions which reduce the cost of healthcare than for the public health strategies designed to care for people and empower disadvantaged sections of the community.

There needs to be a much greater understanding of the total implications of public health, for example in instances such as terrorist attacks, infectious disease outbreaks such as foot and mouth disease or avian flu, or in dealing with effects of global warming, such as flooding. In the broader sense, these examples affect public health in the same way that more individualistic issues such as smoking, obesity and so on, do.

Almost by definition, adults are deemed to be autonomous human beings capable of making decisions for themselves and carrying out actions deriving from those decisions. But in the arena of public health, this may not be the case, or the decisions taken may impact on the health and wellbeing of others. To what extent should decisions taken on a personal level regarding one's own health be revised when considering the health of the community as a whole? Adults might reasonably expect to have the freedom to make their own decisions regarding their health. However, what happens when an individual's wishes conflict with what is in that individual's best interests? Salmon and Omer (2006) suggest that modern public health strives to maximise benefits for the highest number of people while protecting individual rights. Restrictions on individual rights are justified for two reasons – for the benefit of the individual, or the benefit of the community. How far should an individual's rights be restricted for his or her own benefit? In ethical terms, at the very least, this restricts an individual's right to autonomy of decision-making about individual behaviours. Similarly, what limitations should be placed on an individual's behaviour when that person's wishes go against what is good for the population in general? Looker and Hallett (2006) suggest a range of potential conflicts between individual-level wants, individual-level health benefits and population-level health benefits, two examples being refusing the MMR vaccine for one's children, thus decreasing 'herd immunity' in the population, and forcing infected individuals to undergo treatment for tuberculosis so that they do not infect others.

Knowledge of health-harming behaviours is widespread amongst adults (and children) in Western civilisations. So what prevents people from avoiding these? Reasons include an individual's health beliefs, social environment, poverty and poor housing. Kendall (2007) suggests these factors are a major cause of the nine-year difference in life expectancy between men in Manchester and men is Chelsea, London (for instance). Therefore is it more important for government policy to address environmental, educational and other issues than 'preaching' or trying to legislate for the individual lifestyle message? Jenkins (2007) suggests that the smoking ban is a classic example of the government meddling in personal behaviour, while ignoring forms of social control such as family and local self-discipline. On the other hand, governments are accountable, under international human rights treaties, for progressively correcting conditions that may impede realisation of the 'right to health' (Braveman and Gruskin, 2003). This may include tobacco control.

The government wants the smoking rate to fall to 21 per cent by 2010, from 24 per cent in 2007. It has raised the legal age for buying tobacco from 16 to 18. And Sir Liam Donaldson, the Chief Medical Officer, has made no secret of the fact that he would like the ban on smoking to extend further, into people's homes (*Guardian* leader 3 July 2007a). The same article suggests that Britain appears to be moving into an era where people cede choice and accept greater intervention in their personal lives; not so much the return of the nanny state as the coming of the au pair state: a more informal, less heavy-handed but still intrusive creature.

Recent research in Scotland indicates a marked fall in coronary heart disease, for example, since the ban on cigarettes was introduced there (BBC News, 10 September 2007). This adds to the overt message to everyone, smokers and non-smokers, that smoking is unacceptable. The message has been translated from the subtle, to a cultural pervasion of the unacceptability of this behaviour. It has been noted that, in spite of the threat to people's autonomy, there have been very few marked protests against the ban in public places.

There are assumptions that people have the knowledge and resources to 'self-help' in order to make lifestyle changes, such as smoking cessation, but the reality is that barriers can include lack of knowledge, or broader structural issues such as poverty, leading to lack of power, and there are specific groups of people, such as some of those with mental health problems, who depend on smoking as a way of coping with everyday life. There is also the fact that tobacco is itself a very addictive drug, and it can require more resources than just human motivation and willpower to succeed in withdrawing. This means that smokers who are unable, for whatever reason, to stop feel increasingly victimised. This is likely to make smokers light up more at home, leading to role-modelling and passive smoking risks for their children and potentially making things worse for future generations.

The King's Fund in 2004 investigated the public's attitude to public health policy, and found strong support for measures that inform and advise, warn about health risks, and encourage health promotion in the workplace. 'Enabling' measures that help create favourable environmental, economic and social conditions were also strongly supported, particularly by lower socio-economic groups. Support for 'restrictive' measures that try to prevent individuals putting their own or others' health at risk was less. As the report concludes, this indicates clearly that a level of sensitivity is required when public health policy is devised. The practical application of public health needs to be perceived as a concept in which every adult should be involved. Whether this is from a personal viewpoint, or from a more altruist community perspective, public health should be seen as everyone's remit.

CASE STUDY

Government policy and legislation distinguishes between illegal behaviour (for example, drink driving) and behaviour where there are choices – for example, taking exercise. Government policy in the UK recently banned smoking in public places, such as pubs, restaurants, and any other public arena. The 'right' to smoke had gradually become eroded over the last few years prior to the ban, and public opinion has gradually veered from acceptance (or even expectation) of public smoking to treating smokers as pariahs (Bakewell, 2004). Government intervention has proceeded along a gradual, but persistent line, from banning advertising of cigarettes to the now total ban in public places indoors. There is also a proposed plan to put pictures of diseased lungs on cigarette packets to further deter people from smoking, and a proposal to ban cigarette vending machines. But is this a nanny state or a therapeutic state (Fitzpatrick, 2004)?

FURTHER READING

Hunter, D. J. (2003) *Public Health Policy*. Cambridge: Polity Press.
Kelly, A. and Symonds, A. (2003) *The Social Construction of Community Nursing*. Basingstoke: Macmillan.
Wood-Harper, J. (2005) 'Informing education policy on MMR: balancing individual freedoms and collective responsibilities for the promotion of public health', *Nursing Ethics*, 12(1): 43–58.

public health and adults

47 Student Health

Walid El Ansari

KEY POINTS

- It is important to understand students' health in order to tailor health promotion programmes for this population.
- Body weight challenges, nutrition, body shape perceptions and satisfaction and with possible resultant obesity or underweight related to physical activity, mental health, and other burdens due to study are amongst the important health challenges that students face.
- Smoking and alcohol consumption patterns require attention.
- Policies for student health and healthy universities need to address the interlacing nature of the challenges.

DISCUSSION

There are many features that make students an important group whose lifestyle features should be researched as well as health-promoting behaviours, psychological wellbeing or attitudes that are not conducive to health. Firstly most are young adults and the attitudes and lifestyle habits (e.g. smoking, alcohol consumption and physical activity) they adopt during university are likely to affect their lifelong behaviours (Steptoe et al., 2002). Along their lifespan, today's students might function as tomorrow's multipliers of lifestyle behaviours to their extended families and surrounding communities. In some countries, being able to attend study at university or college level is a privilege; hence students make up an educated group that are likely to occupy future administrative and leadership positions. In addition, students are accessible and are likely to participate in studies since many are aware of the importance of research (El Ansari et al., 2007b). In terms of cross-country comparisons, as health and health behaviours are subject to demographic factors, the study of individual country effects can be better disentangled in a group characterised by restricted variations in education, socio-economic status, and age, making students an attractive sample (Stock et al., 2003). The health perceptions of elderly populations have received attention, but less is known about the predictors of self-perceived health in young populations. Unsurprisingly, recent initiatives (e.g. WHO's Health Promoting University Project) affirm that more research is needed in order to guide effective health education and health promotion programmes in the higher education sector. Outlined below are some of the challenges.

Weight challenges, nutrition, and body shape perceptions: obesity and underweight

Obesity is an important risk factor for many diseases, including cardiovascular disease, diabetes and some cancers. It is associated with increased mortality. Adolescent obesity is linked to adulthood obesity (Goodman et al., 2000), so it is a major public health concern. There is lack of research on predictors of and interventions for reducing BMI gain among college students (Adams and Rini, 2007). Recently, there have been suggestions that small-group seminar educational/behavioural intervention successfully prevents weight gain in normal-weight young healthy university students (Hivert et al., 2007).

On the other hand, while the prevalence of obesity is steadily rising, dieting is also increasing, mostly among young women. Dieting during adolescence could herald upcoming eating disorders, given the high dissatisfaction with body weight and body shape in adolescents from industrialised populations.

Physical activity

Physical exercise is key aspects of lifestyle that influences the risk of major diseases such as coronary heart disease. However, it has been shown in many countries awareness of the influence of physical exercise on heart disease is low, ranging between 45 and 50 per cent of men and women (Steptoe et al., 2002). Physical activity is under-studied in college settings, although it has been shown that vigorous physical activity declines from high school to college (Nelson et al., 2007), and social disparities in such activity emerge in college.

The health and financial costs of physical inactivity are staggering. Given that the prevalence of physical activity maintenance in university students is low, and that insufficient physical activity may lead to serious health concerns, interventions are needed to improve activity maintenance in this population. Despite these findings, little research has been conducted on factors that contribute to exercise enjoyment.

Mental health

Anxiety and depression are the commonest challenges to students' mental health: students are more likely to suffer mental health problems because they are concerned about their studies (Wardle et al., 2004). Hence, universities represent an appropriate context for studying youth mental health. Such students often undergo role transitions, for example living away from the family home for the first time, residing with other students, and having reduced adult supervision – changes that might increase the risk of depression.

Mikolajczyk et al. (2007) reported depressive symptoms in student populations from two Eastern and two Western European countries, where a large proportion of students had modified Beck depression inventory (M-BDI) scores equal or above the cut-off point for screening for clinically relevant depression in general population samples. Recent reports from the Royal College of Psychiatrists suggest that students were 1.64 times more likely to experience symptoms of mental ill health than other young people (Harrison, 1999). From small colleges to large universities, the number of college students in distress has grown, with increasing reports of deaths due to substance abuse, homicide and suicide among college students.

Smoking and alcohol

Cigarette smoking is a major health problem among college students, with many students identifying themselves as smokers. Smoking can be associated with poor eating, low physical activity, or negative cardiovascular outcomes. Smoking initiation is higher in girls who diet, suggesting a relationship to body shape satisfaction. Indeed, with heightened attention to body shape and appearance in university-aged students, smoking as an intervention against weight gain is not uncommon.

Similarly, for many students, alcohol consumption is an important aspect of college experience. Heavy drinking is likely to be accompanied by negative outcomes. These include physical harm due to impaired judgement or physical agility caused by alcohol intoxication; unplanned sexual activity; and sexual activity without adequate protection against pregnancy and sexually transmitted diseases. Drinking behaviour is complex. Earlier studies on drinking among college men reported that parental norms, religious traditions and fraternity affiliation were all important normative influences. Other factors play a role in alcohol use: the individual characteristics of drinkers (e.g. gender, residence, importance of college activities) and situational factors (e.g. location, group size, companions). These suggest the need to study a wide range of issues, extending the analysis to the economic, political and ecological factors that have thus far received far less study than the psychosocial issues.

Other burdens

Subjective health and pain complaints are public health problems. Adolescents report headache, backache, musculoskeletal pain and psychological complaints (e.g. nervousness and lack of concentration). Such complaints have economic, health and treatment/medication consequences. For instance, fatigue and low back pain are common among students, and could herald a chronic state to come.

Policies for healthy students/universities

Many factors need to be considered. On the one hand, relationships are intermingled and reciprocal: depressed mood is associated with cigarette smoking, lack of physical exercise, alcohol consumption and sometimes with unhealthy nutrition (Patton et al., 1998). Conversely, absence of smoking, perceived weight and consumption of fruit were independent predictors of physical activity (Seo et al., 2007).

On the other hand, the biological and psychosocial changes experienced by young adults involve bodily experiences and changes in health perceptions. Major diseases of adult life have a behavioural component. Hence it is critical to monitor the trends in young people's health behaviour in order to understand the risk awareness and beliefs that might impact on their uptake of healthy behaviour/s (Steptoe et al., 2002). Suggestions have also been made that gender differences be incorporated in behavioural change programmes geared towards improving awareness of the consequences of lifestyle choices (Dawson et al., 2007).

CASE STUDY: THE CROSS-NATIONAL STUDENT HEALTH STUDY RESEARCH CONSORTIUM

Between 1996 and 2006, universities from seven European countries participated in research on student health behaviours and lifestyles. In three countries (Germany, Spain and Lithuania), a second survey was undertaken about three or four years after the initial baseline survey, following up particular student cohorts. This is important, to detect any trends in students' risk-taking or health-conducive behaviours and health-promoting practices. Some universities collected some objective measurements in addition to surveying the students' health attitudes and behaviours. In 2006 universities from the United Kingdom joined in the research, and currently the consortium is establishing dialogues with new potential partners (Czeck Republic, Slovenia, Egypt) in order to expand the geographical regions that are participating in this collaborative initiative. Such activities will be useful in generating larger datasets, which will reflect student health behaviours in more countries. The consortium has the advantage of increasing the size and diversity of the potential study population, as well as variation in their risk-taking practices or risk-averting lifestyles. However, working in consortia and partnership has many challenges (El Ansari et al., 2007a, 2007b).

CONCLUSION

Clearly a lot of work is still to be undertaken in relation to students' health. The risk factors intertwine and need to be thoroughly understood and disentangled. Only then can specifically tailored, effective, evidence-based health promotion programmes be targeted at this group.

FURTHER READING

Steptoe, A., Wardle, J., Cui, W., Bellisle, F., Zotti, A.M., Baranyai, R. and Sanderman, R. (2002) 'Trends in smoking, diet, physical exercise, and attitudes toward health in European university students from 13 countries, 1990–2000', *Preventive Medicine*, 35 (2): 97–104.

Stock, C., Kücük N., Miseviciene, I., Guillen-Grima, F., Petkeviciene, J. and Aguinaga-Ontoso, I. (2003) 'Differences in health complaints among university students from three European countries', *Preventive Medicine*, 37(6 Pt 1): 535–43.

48 Public Health and the Older Person

Irene Cooke and Jean Mannix

DEFINITION

The term 'older person' is frequently used indiscriminately within health and social care environments, however there appears to be no agreed consensus in defining who the 'older person' in society actually is. This contested issue has raised a number of interesting responses. Ebrahim (2005) indicates that there is a growing international agreement that only those aged 65 and over should be defined as 'elderly'. The Department of Health (2001c) however has identified three separate categories of older person:

1 *Entering old age* – which adopts a socially constructed perspective of those who have completed their career in paid employment and/or child-rearing. Usually aged between 50 years and the official retirement ages of 60 for women and 65 for men.
2 *Transitional phase* – which relates to the transition between healthy, active life and frailty, and usually occurs during the ages of 70–80-plus years, but can occur at any stage of older age.
3 *Frail older people* – which defines those who are vulnerable as a result of health problems such as stroke or dementia, social care needs or a combination of both. Usually aged over 80 years.

Consequently, when reviewing the concept of public health and the older person, it is important to recognise that older people are a heterogeneous population, comprising those who are independently pursuing careers, those who are actively enjoying retirement, those who are caring for family members, including partners and grandchildren, and finally others who are frail and dependent upon others (Ebrahim, 2005). Therefore, older people experience diverse and complex personal, social and healthcare needs that span a continuum from marginal to intensive need requirements (Reed et al., 2007). This very dissimilar population group requires interventions which meet all of their health and social care needs both sensitively and comprehensively.

KEY POINTS

- The older population are a heterogeneous group who experience diverse and varied health and social care needs.
- The older population are the most frequent users of the NHS.
- The risks and consequences of disease can be reduced or their onset delayed by lifestyle modifications.
- Maintaining the health of the older population optimises older people's contribution to society.
- Health inequalities exist in older population groups.

DISCUSSION

The world is ageing. Internationally, people are living longer than ever before and the number of older people is increasing, both worldwide and in the United Kingdom (WHO, 2004; NSO, 2004). This translates into the current picture of one in six people in the population being aged 65 or over (Age Concern, 2006b). It is projected that by 2050, there will be more people aged 60 and over than children under the age of 15 (WHO, 2004). This demographic shift will have significant implications for society and the utilisation of healthcare services both now and in the future.

The study of older people and public health has primarily focused on two main areas: (a) The concept of wellbeing, and (b) the morbidity of ill health, which we will now explore.

Concept of wellbeing

Although the life expectancy of older people has increased, this does not necessarily mean that they will experience worse health (Fitzpatrick, 2001). When Age Concern (2006b) conducted a survey of older people, they discovered that older people were generally knowledgeable about what is required to maintain health, and that they view health holisti-cally with an intuitive understanding of healthy ageing. They also found that older people defined a healthy lifestyle as one which included having a positive frame of mind, a balanced diet, an active lifestyle, mental stimulation and social contact. Other studies have indicated that feeling autonomous, retaining identity and feeling that life has meaning and is worthwhile are also important factors which the older population feel contribute to wellbeing (JRF, 2005; Bryant et al., 2001) and to the quality of life experienced.

It is therefore important to recognise that when targeting health and social interventions at older populations, the professional needs to work in partnership with the individual or client group to identify and acknowledge the health beliefs, values, feelings, attitudes and priorities, which may be predetermined by client groups experiences of health and ill health. These experiences should not be underestimated, as they con-tribute to the evolving partnership between the individual and the health and social care professional. Recognition of these essential factors should enable the setting of more realistic and achievable health and social care goals to maintain health. Also, an interesting finding is that some older people feel that they do not need to change their lifestyle and that their age is testimony to that (Age Concern, 2006b).

A significant aim of public health is to 'increase the period of later life which is free from poor health, incapacity and dependency' (Donaldson and Donaldson, 2003: 364), so the prevention of morbidity and disability rather than mortality may be a more relevant focus for older people (Acheson, 1998). The World Health Organization (2004) has expanded on this theme by defining healthy ageing as 'the process of optimizing opportunities for health, participation and security in order to enhance quality of life as people age'.

Health is a dynamic and evolving process and when considering the quality of life, as opposed to the duration, it is important to determine what the individual or group's concept of wellbeing actually is, so services and support can be structured to encompass their needs, thereby contributing to realistic care delivery and optimal health status.

Morbidity of ill health

As a person ages, their cumulative exposure to environmental and lifestyle risks increases, resulting in a higher probability of developing chronic disease (HM Treasury, 2004) and disability (WHO, 2004). Many elderly people live with varying degrees of poor health and have an enhanced need for health and social care services. Older people who live with long-term conditions such as diabetes may require healthcare interventions to manage their activities of daily living; however, many prefer to stay at home, rather than be admitted to hospital (McKeown, 2007). As older people are the most frequent users of NHS services (DH, 2001c), there will be resource implications for health and social care service providers, to ensure that care is delivered both timely and comprehensively to meet the individuals' needs. There is evidence that identifying a high incidence of hospital readmission among older people may lead to health and social care interventions to enable the individual to remain at home with appropriate support and care (DH, 2003d). It has also been found that the risks and consequences of the disease trajectory can be reduced or their onset delayed by lifestyle modifications in many cases (Age Concern, 2006a).

An interesting finding relates to the Joseph Rowntree Foundation (2005), which identified that older people want help which will enable them to remain as independent as possible, and frequently minimal support is required to maximise independence. This indicates that many older people are able to lead independent lifestyles with minimal intervention from professional groups, as opposed to requiring complex health and social care support. Multi-professional care should therefore aim to be supportive in maximising opportunities for individuals to achieve their desired goals and outcomes rather than focusing only upon medical approaches to health deficits and challenges.

There are factors which can contribute to the overall wellbeing and morbidity of older people living in a community. It is reported that fear about the neighbourhood and potential crime can affect whether older people will go out of their homes (NWPHO, 2002). As well as affecting an individual's physical health status by limiting opportunities for mobilisation and exercise, the individuals' mental health and wellbeing may also be compromised and social isolation become the normal pattern within a community. Such events may lead to increased levels of depression and anxiety being reported (NWPHO, 2002; Runciman et al., 2006).

Finally, it has also been reported that there is an increase in life expectancy amongst older populations from different social strata (Marmot et al., 2002). Inequalities in health affect elderly population groups in that there are differences in health experienced according to socio-economic status (Asthana and Halliday, 2006). This is a significant finding, and indicates that whilst health inequalities exist within both the older population and the rest of society, they also exist within the older population as a subgroup in itself. Societal and government agencies have a key responsibility to prioritise older people's health and wellbeing, in order to proactively meet the needs of the changing demographic shift and to give due cognisance to the healthy ageing agenda.

CASE STUDY

Janet is a community nurse working in a busy urban area and her case-load comprises a number of older people, who have been referred to the community nurse for the management of long-term conditions. Janet recently undertook a health needs profile of her practice population, and found that a significant number of the older population are regularly readmitted to the local hospital for short-term health interventions, and then discharged back home. Following a review of each individual case, Janet decided that a proactive, rather than a reactive approach would be required to maximise the health potential of each individual in order to prevent readmission. While in partnership with the older person, Janet worked closely with the multi-professional team and other statutory and voluntary agencies, such as housing and social services, and through the clinical governance agenda was able to organise appropriate social and healthcare support for the individuals concerned. Education and advice regarding lifestyle choices was offered to those who required it using a health empowerment model, which resulted in the individuals feeling more confident in remaining at home, thereby facilitating a reduced hospital readmission rate.

CONCLUSION

This chapter has explored the concept of public health and older people from a number of perspectives. We have found that the changing demography of the older population presents future challenges for health and social care professionals. It is anticipated that the resources required to maintain older people within the community environment will require considerable investment, on both financial and societal levels, in an attempt to address some of the health inequalities which exist.

FURTHER READING

Marmot, M., Banks, J., Blundell, R., Lessof, C. and Nazroo, J. (2002) *Health, Wealth and Lifestyles of the Older Population in England: The 2002 English Longitudinal Study of Ageing*. London: Institute for Fiscal Studies.

Themessl-Huber, M., Hubbard, G. and Munro, P. (2007) 'Frail older people's experiences and use of health and social care services', *Journal of Nursing Management* (15): 222–9.

49 Public Health and Homelessness

Judith Lydon and Scott Harrison

DEFINITION

According to English law, a person is homeless if they have no accommodation that they are entitled to occupy or they have accommodation but it is not reasonable for them to continue occupying it (DCLG, 1996). There are wider definitions of homelessness including 'rough sleeping' and 'sofa-surfing', but the legal definition relates to the right to a home, not the circumstances in which someone lacks a home (SEU, 1998). It is important to note that homelessness is also often interpreted as the lack of suitable accommodation – if a person is housed in substandard accommodation, they may be classed by some service providers as 'functionally homeless' as the accommodation does not meet basic requirements for health, safety and security.

KEY POINTS

- Homelessness is a growing concern in many Western countries, including the United Kingdom (Shinn, 2007).

- Homelessness is often the result of complex socio-economic factors and has lasting consequences on the health of both affected individuals and the wider community (Lee et al., 2003).
- Homelessness and poverty are inextricably linked. The cost of accommodation often absorbs a high proportion of income. People living in poverty are frequently unable to pay for housing, food, education or healthcare.
- Addressing homelessness is challenging for social policy makers due to the multi-dimensionality of the issue (Roche, 2004). Homelessness is intrinsically linked to systems of social welfare, public housing policies, employment patterns and, increasingly, shifts in global migration.
- Homeless people are often socially excluded and marginalised. The act of marginalization further compounds the myriad health and social problems already faced by the homeless.
- Public health workers are ideally placed to develop policies which seek to address and overcome the issues of access and inclusion for homeless people.

DISCUSSION

Social policy in the United Kingdom has shifted in recent years towards addressing the complex social and health issues related to homelessness and the asylum and refugee processes (SEU, 1998). Homelessness is a growing public health issue in the UK. This has arisen both as a response to real and identifiable need – in particular the evidence of increasing numbers of homeless people and asylum applicants and the allied consequences of this for service provision – and as a result of broader trends and issues including the growing number of people living in poverty.

Biomedical theories that often guide the work of health services do not explain the health impact of these social issues, which often have negative health consequences. A clear example of this can be found in homelessness, which has significant consequences for both individuals and the wider community. Homeless people and asylum applicants experience poorer levels of general physical and mental health than the general population and there is a substantial international evidence base which documents multiple morbidity. Despite this, they often have problems in obtaining suitable healthcare.

Social exclusion is a central factor of homelessness – people without a home are often forced into temporary accommodation or a life on the streets, which carries multiple risks for health and wellbeing. Inadequate shelter, food and access to healthcare are compounded by a transitory lifestyle, where the primary goal becomes survival rather than wellbeing. The foundation of public health nursing is the promotion of human rights and social justice, which makes public health nurses excellent advocates for challenging poverty, homelessness and social exclusion (Falk-Rafael, 2005).

Cohen and Reutter (2007) identify considerable theoretical, historical and professional support for the role of public health nurses in addressing and reducing the impact of child and family poverty, which remains intrinsically linked to homelessness and social exclusion. Central to this role is the engagement of individuals, communities and other services in the development of services and policies which address both the immediate problems of homelessness and the social causes of the issue. The key to effective public health nursing interventions with homeless clients is collaboration – with both the individual or family and the existing service providers and community partners.

CASE STUDY

A young man aged 19 had been a rough sleeper for the past year. He was placed into care at age 12 by his family, due to complex behavioural problems and the family's inability to cope. Up until he left care, he was generally well and did not require long-term care or medication; however, his health deteriorated rapidly once he entered into a life on the streets. Staff at the local night shelter contacted the public health nurse as they were becoming concerned that his behaviour was on occasions erratic and odd – this would sometimes last up to five hours.

The public health nurse met with the client and completed a full health assessment. This uncovered information about a new signifying practice in street-involved youth in the town: the injection of blood into each other's veins in order to become 'blood brothers'. This was having dangerous consequences as this young man was putting himself at high risk of blood-borne diseases and was suffering the effects of the drug-taking practices of his 'blood brothers'.

The public health nurse pulled together a multi-agency meeting to discuss the practice and find out more about the experiences of other service providers in the town. As a result, a number of health education sessions were held at the local night shelter, the local day centre and various hostels for the homeless.

The public health nurse also held informal focus groups with the core members of this blood brotherhood to explore perceptions and attitudes to this practice and the information gained in these meetings was used to promote 'safer' behaviours, reduce risk and ultimately discourage the practice altogether. The public health nurse determined from these focus groups that the impact of social exclusion and a poor sense of community were key factors in the development of the blood brotherhood. She supported the group to advocate for improved access to day centres and night shelters, so the group could socialise more and feel more connected to the community.

CONCLUSION

Public health nurses are ideally placed to support homeless people both on the individual level and also on a wider community level, by engaging service providers and communities to consider ways in which the causes and impacts of homelessness can be addressed and negated. For individuals, our principal role should be engagement and increasing access to both preventive services and treatment programmes for existing health problems. Public health nurses often have extensive knowledge and experience of their local community and can assist in linking homeless people to existing services and working as advocates where services are required but do not yet exist.

FURTHER READING

Curtis, S. (2004) *Health and Inequality*. London: Sage.

Lee, B.A., Price-Spratlen, T. and Kanan, J.W. (2003) 'Determinants of homelessness in metropolitan areas', *Journal of Urban Affairs*, 25(3): 335–56.

Roche, M. (2004) 'Complicated problems, complicated solutions? Homelessness and joined up policy responses', *Social Policy and Administration*, 38(7): 758–74.

public health and homelessnes

50 Public Health in the Workplace

Alan Massey

DEFINITION

In *Making a Difference*, (DH, 1999b) the Department of Health encourages occupational health nurses to expand their role by adopting a broader public health approach, emphasising the importance of improving health and tackling inequalities. This expanded role was highlighted in the DH (2003a) document, *Taking a Public Health Approach in the Workplace*. It defined public health in the workplace as,

> Working to improve the quality of life for everyone in the workforce and involving people in the wider issues that affect health. This can be done through partnership working, engaging with different groups and communities and encouraging people to participate in the decisions about their health. (2003a: 6)

The format for achievement was made clear in 2004 via the strategy for the Health and Wellbeing of Working Age People, which highlighted that occupational health practitioners must; (a) engage with stakeholders; (b) improve working lives by proactively minimising the risk of employees becoming ill, improving employee retention by supporting them during periods of transition and building a workplace that rehabilitates rather than rejects people with illness or disability; and (c) provide appropriate healthcare for people in the workplace based on an assessment of need (DH, 2004c).

KEY POINTS

- Health inequalities should be addressed in the workplace.
- Collaborative working is essential in the development of occupational health provision.
- The workplace is a key setting in which to address health.
- Service provision should be based on an assessment of need.

DISCUSSION

The workplace is an environment in which full-time employees may spend 50 per cent of their waking time, and it influences health primarily by factors contained within the environment that are detrimental to or enhance health and by the process of work itself (Taylor et al., 2004). The workplace is known to have inherent 'risks' to health, such as physical, chemical, biological and psychological factors. The identification, elimination/control, and monitoring of risks to health in the workplace is essential in ensuring that work does not have a detrimental effect.

Harris (2005) and Tones and Tilford (2001) highlight a paradoxical relationship between work and health. Work is considered to be intrinsically good for human beings and there is a wealth of evidence to support the view that unemployment has a greater detrimental effect on health than work. However, this argument is countered by the knowledge that people die or are made ill from work. The Health and Safety Executive (HSE) produce yearly statistics, which highlight the extent of the problem:

- 2.2 million people were suffering from an illness they believed was caused or made worse by work.
- 241 workers were killed while at work, with 141,350 injuries reported via RIDDOR.
- 36 million days were lost due to work-related illness or injury.

(HSE, 2007)

Work is acknowledged as one of the key determinates of health (WHO, 2005). Much of its significance lies in the socio-economic benefits that, for example, financial stability provides (Fleming, 2007). Consideration should be given to the type of work undertaken as, according to Marmot and Wilkinson (2001), those undertaking menial jobs with little or no control will suffer greater ill health caused by work than their superiors who have a degree of control and direction. Thus, the health inequalities of our early socialisation can be perpetuated and it is a public health imperative that health inequalities be removed. The aim is to reduce health inequalities and the burden of morbidity and mortality; and to create healthy workplaces which are more productive, efficient and environmentally safe and which empower and value all stakeholders (Watterson, 2003).

Addressing public health in the workplace and engaging stakeholders

The rationale for addressing health in the workplace is clear. In seeking to deal with the workplace within a public health remit, understanding of the premise that health is created in the relationship between individuals and their environments (i.e the settings in which they live, work and play) is required (Ottawa Charter, WHO, 1986). Tones and Tilford (2001) and Watterson (2003) indicate that the workplace is a challenging environment in which to undertake public health. This is due to the differing needs of the key stakeholders and the inherent power imbalance in many workplaces. This leads to the dominance of employers' values over the values of the other stakeholders. According to Waldron (1980) the value set for employers is an economic one, for the health professional it is wellbeing focused, and for the employees it is a mix of both of these elements. Fleming (2007) indicates that a healthy workplace can be achieved if shared values are developed in an inclusive, facilitative environment which adheres to the principles of equity, empowerment, respect and informed participation. These principles now underline HSE strategies, such as Worker Involvement in Health and Safety Management (HSE, 2004), which provides examples of how these factors can be incorporated. The principles dictate the need for a healthy, qualified and motivated workforce to deal with the risks faced in the modern workplace. This knowledge has led to an increased understanding that employers must seek to address the multi-determinates of people's health via a sociological or whole systems approach. Successful public health approaches lie in achieving shared goals for health improvements via the interested stakeholders, incorporating factors that are economically and socially productive and that are empowering rather than constraining. Oakley (2002) provides us with a framework for understanding the key stakeholders in her discussion on assessing the organisation so that business and health goals can become mutually compatible (see Box 50.1). Within this process consensus can be reached so that occupational health services are developed which address the systems that are present within organisations and that affect health.

272

Box 50.1

- Identify key personnel
- Identify the structure and demographics of the organisation
- Obtain sickness absence policies and procedures

- Determine current pre-employment procedures
- Conduct a site visit
- Assess exposure to health hazards
- Assess compliance with health and safety legislation
- Assess first aid facilities
- Obtain details of compensation claims against the organisation over the past ten years.
- Determine expectations of managers and employees for an occupational health service.

Source: Oakley (2002)

O'Donnell (2002) points out that public health approaches have been slow to develop due to the dominance of the biomedical model of healthcare. O'Donnell's research indicates that biomedical approaches are expensive and have minimal impact and that by focusing on those who already have disease or who undertake risky health behaviours are counterproductive. His research shows that a whole systems approach to assessing the workplace, including risk assessments and health needs analysis, is cost-effective. Fleming (2007) supports this and highlights an emerging body of knowledge from organisations such as the European Network of Health Promoting Workplaces that can be utilised to demonstrate the economic and social benefits of whole systems approaches to employers and other interested stakeholders. This evidence will also ensure that the priorities set will have resonance with the employers and employees, thus addressing the needs of all key stakeholders.

In seeking to improve the working lives of the workplace community, the Nursing and Midwifery Council (NMC) indicates that public health practice involves four public health 'domains': these are further divided into principles for practice, which inform the public health practitioner of their role (see Box 50.2).

Box 50.2 Standards of proficiency for specialist community public health nursing

- Search for health needs
- Stimulation of awareness of health needs
- Influence on policies affecting health
- Facilitation of health enhancing activities

Source: NMC (2004)

public health in the workplace

These elements can be incorporated into occupational health practice utilising primary secondary and tertiary approaches to service provision (see Figure 50.1).

In assessing the above roles it is clear that occupational health is a complex multi-professional undertaking and that the successful development of effective service provision must be inclusive, proactive and evidence based.

Improving working lives by minimising risk

As we have seen, the workplace can be an unsafe environment. Specific protection is the duty of all present in the workplace. Responsibilities for health and safety are laid out in the Health and Safety at Work Act [HSWA] 1974. This is usually achieved via the process of risk assessment. Since the introduction of the HSWA organisations have focused mainly on addressing the hazardous physical conditions that exist in the workplace (Taylor et al., 2004). This has led to the dominance of safety over health. However, the world of work has changed significantly since the Act's inception and the risk factors present in the modern workplace may not be physical in nature. The occupational practitioner should seek to influence the risk assessment process in greater detail by highlighting the effects of hazards to health. The process should focus on assisting the employer to meet their statutory requirements, ensuring that the workplace is non-detrimental to health and creating a healthy and supportive environment. Analysing factors such as the work/life balance, safe systems of work, addressing health behaviours etc. can lead to the creation of a more productive, healthier workforce.

Provision of service and rehabilitation

If we accept the premise that work is good for us then we need to understand that we must do all we can to assist people to remain in work or to help them return to work. Provision of service should be organised via an organisational assessment and via a health needs assessment to ensure tailored services. Rehabilitation should be structured around the concept of early intervention and supportive environments (Taylor et al., 2004). Early intervention strategies are known to be effective in reducing sickness absence (HSE, 2004a). Rehabilitation should be designed to get people back to work as soon as possible after they become ill, and managing absence effectively from day one. Effective systems which manage communication between health service providers, employees and employers is crucial in the development of appropriate

Primary prevention
Health needs assessments
Organisational assessment
Health promotion/health education
Compliance with legislation
Programme development/improving working practices/standards/policies for behavioural risks (nutrition, no smoking, etc.) via effective collaboration and communication
Planning, design and maintenance of equipment and substances used at work
Promoting the adaptation of work to the worker
Collaboration in training and education in occupational health, hygiene and ergonomics
Attention to personality development/awareness of psychological issues, personal risk assessments/empowerment and skills development
Provision of adequate recreation, and working conditions
Counselling
Structured and periodic screening
Quality enhancement programmes

Specific protection
Use of the specific immunisations (influenza, etc.)
Attention to personal hygiene/infection control
Use of environmental monitoring/hygiene/ergonomics
Protection against occupational hazards (organisational risk assessments)
Protection from accidents
Protection from carcinogens (environmental monitoring and toxicology)
Risk/safety/waste management

Secondary prevention
Risk identification and management
  (organisational)
Health surveillance (environment)
Health surveillance (personal)
Occupational hygiene, ergonomics and
  personal protective equipment
First aid and emergency treatment
Accident investigation and analysis
Case finding measures: individual and mass
  screening
Sickness absence management/wellness
  attendance

Selective examinations to:
cure and prevent disease process
prevent spread of communicable disease
Prevent complications and sequelae
Period of disability

Disability limitations
Adequate treatment to arrest disease process
  and prevent further complications
Provision of facilities to limit disability and
  prevent death

**Tertiary prevention:
restoration and
rehabilitation**
Vocational rehabilitation
Provision of hospital and community
  facilities for retraining and
  education to maximise use of
  remaining capacities.
Education of public and industry
  to use rehabilitated persons to
  fullest possible extent
Selective placement
Work therapy in hospitals
Use of sheltered accommodation/
  work

public health in the workplace

Figure 50.1 *Primary, secondary and tertiary approaches to occupational health practice*

care. Occupational health providers should look at implementing or buying in services with a known evidence base, which may delay rehabilitation if provided by the National Health Service or the private sector: for example physiotherapy. The practitioner should also be knowledgeable of the workers' compensation system in order to protect both the employer and the employee and inform them of their statutory rights. Finally, the occupational health service should seek to provide targeted and structured health promotion to allow clients to make healthier choices.

CASE STUDY

A public health approach commences with a health needs assessment: this includes identifying the organisational commitment to addressing health. Once the health needs of your workforce have been identified they can be dealt with in a systematic and cost-effective manner by prioritisation and by taking a whole systems approach. This must be achieved by participation of all stakeholders. Steering groups are useful mechanisms in achieving this aim. Consultation must occur and results from the consultation process must be included in the organisational health plan. Implementation strategies should take a bottom up approach so that ownership of the health plan remains with the organisation as a whole. Evaluation of your initiatives should be conducted on a regular basis to ensure aims and objectives are met.

FURTHER READING

Department of Health (2004a) *Health, Work and Wellbeing: A Strategy for the Health and Wellbeing of Working Age People.* London: DH.
Department of Health (2004b) *Taking a Public Health Approach in the Workplace.* London: DH.
Scriven, A. and Garmen, S. (2007) *Public Health: Social Context and Action.* London: McGraw-Hill.

Acheson, D. (1998) *Independent Inquiry into Inequalities in Health Report*. London: Stationery Office.

Adams, T. and Rini, A. (2007) 'Predicting 1-year change in body mass index among college students', *Journal Am. Coll. Health*, 55(6): 361–5.

Aday, L. (1993) *The Health and Healthcare Needs of Vulnerable Populations in the United States*. San Francisco: Jossey Bass.

Adshead, F., Thorpe, A. and Rutter, J. (2006). 'Sustainable development and public health: a national perspective', *Public Health*, 120: 1102–5.

Age Concern (2006a). *'As Fit as Butchers' Dogs?' Report on Healthy Lifestyle Choice and Older People*. Retrieved 12 December 2007, from http:www.ageconcern.org.uk

Age Concern (2006b) *Public Health and Health Inequalities: Position Paper*. Retrieved 5 December 2007, from http://www.ageconcern.org.uk/AgeConcern/health_ policy_ position.asp

Aggleton, P., Blenkinshop, S., Chase, E., Eggers, M., Schagen, I., Schagen, S. et al. (2004) *Evaluation of the Impact of the National Healthy School Standard*. London: National Foundation for Educational Research/ Thomas Coram Research Unit.

Albee, G. W. and Ryan-Finn, K. (1993) 'An overview of primary prevention', *Journal of Counselling and Development*, 72: 115–23.

Alexander, M. P., Zakocs, R. C., Earp, J. A. and French, E. (2006) 'Community coalition project directors: what makes them effective leaders?' *Journal of Public Health Management and Practice*, 2(2): 201–9.

Andersson, E., Tritter, J. and Wilson, R. (2006) *Healthy Democracy: The Future of Involvement in Health and Social Care*. London: Involve/NCI.

Andreasen, A. R. (2002) 'Marketing social marketing in the social change marketplace', *Journal of Public Policy and Marketing*, 21: 3–13.

APHO (Association of Public Health Observatories) (2005) *Indications of Public Health in the English Regions 4: Ethnicity and Health*. London: APHO.

Armstrong, D. (1993). 'From clinical gaze to a regime of total' *Health Education Journal*, 52(3): 114–19.

Armstrong, D. (1995) 'The rise of surveillance medicine', *Sociology of Health and Illness*, 17(3): 393–404.

Aronson, J. K. (2007) 'Compliance, concordance, adherence', *British Journal of Clinical Pharmacology*, 63(4): 383–4.

Ashton, A. and Seymour, H. (1992) *The New Public Health*. Milton Keynes: Open University Press.

Association of Public Health Observatories (2005) *Indications of Public Health in the English Regions 4: Ethnicity and Health*. London: APHO.

Asthana, S. and Halliday, J. (2006) *What Works in Tackling Health Inequalities? Pathways, Policies and Practice through the Lifecourse*. Bodmin: Policy Press.

Atkins, C. and Louw, G. (2000) 'Reclaiming knowledge: a case for evidence based information systems'. Paper presented at the European Conference on Information Systems.

Australia. State of the Environment Committee (2001) *Australian State of the Environment 2001: Independent Report to the Commonwealth Minister for the Environment and Heritage.* Retrieved 10 December 2007, from http://www.environment.gov.au/soe/2001/publications/report/index.html

Baggott, R. (2000) *Public Health: Policy and Politics.* Basingstoke: Palgrave Macmillan.

Baker, D., Mead, N. and Cambell, S. (2002) 'Inequalities in morbidity and consulting behaviour for socially vulnerable groups', *British Journal of General Practice,* 52(475): 124–30.

Bakewell, J. (2004) *Just70.* Retrieved 23 July 2007, from http://society.guardian.co.uk/health/comment

Bandolier (2000) 'What is critical appraisal'. Retrieved 20 March 2007, from www.medicine.ox.ac.uk/bandolier/painres/download/whatis/What_is_critical_appraisal.pdf

Bandura, A. (1986) *Social Foundations of Thought and Action. A Social Cognitive Theory.* Englewood Cliffs, NJ: Prentice-Hall.

Barlow, J., Turner, A. P. and Wright, C. C. (2000) *Self-management Literature Review.* Coventry: Coventry University.

Barnes, R., Nelson, P. and Stanton, J. (2004) *Delivering a New Wembley: Health Impact Assessment.* London: Brent Teaching Primary Care Trust.

Barton, J. and Parry-Jones, W. (2004) 'Adolescence', in R. Detels, J. McEwan, R. Beaglehole and H. Tanaka (eds) *Oxford Textbook of Public Health,* 4th edn. Oxford: Oxford University Press. pp. 1623–38.

BBC News (2007) *Scots Smoke Ban 'Improved Health'.* Retrieved 10 December 2007, from http://news.bbc.co.uk/1/hi/scotland/edinburgh_and_east/6986554.stm

Beaglehole, R. (2004) 'Determinants of health and disease: overview and framework', in R. Detels, J. McEwan, R. Beaglehole and H. Tanaka (eds), *Oxford Textbook of Public Health,* 4th edn. Oxford: Oxford University Press.

Beaglehole, R. and Bonita, R. (1997) 'Reinvigorating public health', *Lancet,* 56(9232): 787–8.

Beaglehole, R., Bonita, R. and Kjellstron, T. (1993) *Basic Epidemiology.* Geneva: World Health Organization.

Beck, U. (1992) *Risk Society: Towards a New Modernity.* London: Sage.

Beck, U. (1995) *Ecological Politics in an Age of Risk.* Cambridge: Polity Press.

Belbin, R. M. (1993) *Team Roles at Work.* Oxford: Butterworth Heinmann.

Bell, S. J., Airaksinen, M. S., Lyles, A., Chen, T. F. and Aslani, P. (2007) 'Concordance is not synonymous with compliance or adherence' (Letters to the Editor), *British Journal of Clinical Pharmacology,* 64(5): 710–13.

Benenson, A. (1995) *Control of Communicable Diseases Manual,* 16th edn. Washington, DC: American Public Health Association.

Bennett, P. and Calman, K. (1999) *Risk Communication and Public Health.* Oxford: Oxford University Press.

Bentall, P. R. (2003) *Madness Explained: Understanding Psychosis and the Human Condition.* London: Penguin.

Berg, R. (2005a) 'Environmental health and the media, part 1: overcoming shark phobias', *Journal of Environmental Health,* 68(4): 40–9.

Berg, R. (2005b) 'Environmental health and the media, part 2: beyond get the message out/put the fires out', *Journal of Environmental Health,* 68(5): 36–44.

Bergman-Evans, B. (2006) 'AIDES to improving medication adherence in older adults', *Geriatric Nursing*, 27: 174–82.

Bibbings, R. (2007) 'Risk education', *The RoSPA Occupational Safety and Health Journal*, 37(5): 62–3.

Bird, W. (2004) *Natural Fit. Can Green Space and Biodiversity Increase Levels of Physical Activity?* (Royal Society for the Protection of Birds). Retrieved 10 December 2007, from http://www.rspb.org.uk/Images/natural_fit_full_version_tcm9-133055.pdf

Black, D. (1980) *Inequalities in Health: Report of a Research Working Group*. Retrieved 20 August 2007, from http://www.sochealth.co.uk/history/black.htm

Blair, M., Stewart-Brown, S., Waterson, T. and Crowther, R. (2004) *Child Public Health*. Oxford: Oxford University Press.

Blows, W. T. (2003) *The Biological Basis of Nursing: Mental Health*. London: Routledge.

Bolden, R., Gosling, R., Marturano, A. and Dennison, P. (2003) *A Review of Leadership Theory and Competency Frameworks*. Exeter: University of Exeter, Centre for Leadership Studies.

Bongaarts, J. and Griffith, F. (1998) 'On the quantum and tempo of fertility', *Population Fertility Review*, 24(2): 271–91.

Bourdieu, P. (1984) *Distinction: A Social Critique of the Judgement of Taste*. London: Routledge and Kegan Paul.

Boyd, N. R. and Windsor, R. A. (2003) 'Formative evaluation in maternal and child health practice: The partners for life nutrition education program for pregnant women', *Maternal and Child Health Journal*, 7(2): 137–43.

Bradley, P. and Burls, A. (2002) *Ethics in Public and Community Health*. London: Routledge.

Bradshaw, J. (1972) 'The concept of social need', *New Society*, 19(469): 640–2.

Braveman, P. and Gruskin, S. (2003) 'Poverty, equity, human rights and health', *Bulletin of the World Health Organisation*, 81: 7. Retrieved 20 December 2007, from http://www.scielosp.org

Breinbauer, C. and Maddaleno, M. (2005) *Youth Choices and Changes: Promoting Healthy Behaviours in Adolescents*. Washington: WHO.

Bridges, W. (2004) *Transitions: Making Sense of Life's Changes*, 2nd edn. New York: Addison-Wesley.

The British Liver Trust (1999) *Living a Healthy Life with Long Term Illness. The Board of Trustees*. Leland Stanford Junior University: The Board of Trustees.

Bronfenbrenner, U. (1979) *The Ecology of Human Development: Experiments by Nature and Design*. Cambridge, MA: Harvard University Press.

Brown, J., Shassere, E. and Sengupta, S. (2005) *Health in Regional Public Policy: Using Assessment Techniques to Improve the Impact of Policy on Health*. Stockton-on-Tees: Health Development Agency/University of Durham.

Bryant, L. L., Corbett, K. K. and Kutner, J. S. (2001) 'In their own words: a model of healthy aging', *Social Science and Medicine*, 53(7): 927–41.

Brynner, J. (2005) 'Rethinking the youth phase of the life-course: the case for emerging adulthood?', *Journal of Youth Studies*, 8(4): 367–84.

Buchanan, D. R. (2000) *An Ethic for Health Promotion. Rethinking the Sources of Human Wellbeing*. Oxford: Oxford University Press.

Bunton, R., Murphy, S. and Bennet, P. (1991) 'Theories of behaviour change and their use in health promotion: some neglected areas', *Health Education Research*, 6(2): 153–62.

Burgon, C. (2007) 'Introduction to the Expenditure and Food Survey', *Nutrition Bulletin*, 32: 283–6.

Buss, D. (1998) 'Registered Public Health Nutritionist (RPHNutr): a new qualification in public health nutrition.', *Nutrition and Food Science*, 98(3).

Buttriss, J., Stanner, S., McKevith B., Nugent, A. P., Kelly, C., Phillips, K. and Theobald, H. E. (2004) 'Successful ways to modify food choice: lessons from the literature', *Nutrition Bulletin*, 29(4): 333–43.

Cairns, J. (1995) 'The costs of prevention', *British Medical Journal*, 311(1520): 1–5

Caraher, M. Dixon, P., Lang, T. and Carr-Hill, R. (1999) 'The state of cooking in England: The relationship of cooking skills to food choice', *British Food Journal*, 101(8): 590–609.

Carter, N. (2001) 'Understanding sustainable development'. Retrieved 8 February 2008, from http://www.fathom.com/course/21701763/session1.html

Castel, R. (1991) 'From dangerousness to risk', in G. Burchell, C. Gordon and P. Miller (eds), *The Foucault Effect: Studies in Governmentality*. Brighton: Harvester Wheatsheaf.

Casting for Recovery (2008) *Casting for Recovery*. Retrieved 3 April 2008, from http://www.castingforrecovery.org.uk

Cattan, M. (2006) *Mental Health Promotion: A Life Span Approach*. London: Open University.

Caulfield, H. (2006) *Accountability Vital Notes for Nurses*. Oxford: Blackwell.

CCDC in America (2007) *The State of Aging and Health in America 2007*. Retrieved 23 June 2007, from www.cdc.gov/Aging/pdf/saha_2007.pdf

Centers for Disease Control and Prevention (2001) *Updated Guidelines for Evaluating Public Health Surveillance Systems. Recommendations from the Guidelines Working Group. Morbidity and Mortality Weekly Report*. Atlanta, GA: Centre for Disease Control and Prevention.

Centers for Disease Control and Prevention (2002) 'General recommendations on immunization: recommendations of the Advisory Committee on Immunization practices and the American Academy of Family Physicians', *MMWR*, 51(2): 1–2

Centre for Reviews and Dissemination (2001) *CRD Report 4*, 2nd edn. York: CRD.

Centre for Urban and Community Research (2005) *Investors in Communities: Final Evaluation Report on Pilot Phase*. York: Joseph Rowntree Foundation.

Chen, H. T. (2005) *Practical Programme Evaluation*. London: Sage.

Clark, N. and McLeroy, K. (1998) 'Reviewing the evidence for health promotion in the United States', in J. K. Davies and G. Macdonald (eds), *Quality, Evidence and Effectiveness in Health Promotion*. London: Routledge. pp. 21–46.

Cohen, B. E. and Reutter, L. (2007) 'Development of the role of public health nurses in addressing child and family poverty: a framework for action', *Journal of Advanced Nursing*, 60(1), 96–107.

Coleman, J. and Hendry, L. (1999) *The Nature of Adolescence*, 3rd edn. London: Routledge.

COMEAP (2006) *Cardiovascular Disease and Air Pollution. A Report by the Committee on the Medical Effects of Air Pollutants*, chairman, J.G. Ayres. Retrieved 1 August 2007, from http://www.advisorybodies.doh.gov.uk/comeap/statementsreports/CardioDisease.pdf

Cooner, R. F., Tanjasiri, S. P., Dempsey, C. L., Robles, G., Davidson, M. B. and Easterling, D. V. (2003) 'The Colorado Healthy Communities Initiative: Communities defining and addressing health', in D. V. Easterling, K. M. Gallagher and D. G. Lodwick (eds) *Promoting Health at the Community Level*. Thousand Oaks, CA: Sage. pp. 17–24.

Cooper, H. and Geyer, R. (2007) *Riding the Diabetes Rollercoaster: A New Approach for Health Professionals, Patients and Carers*. Oxford: Radcliffe.

Copp, L. A. (1986) 'The nurse as advocate for vulnerable persons', *Journal of Advanced Nursing*, 11: 255–63.

Costello, J. and Haggart, M. (2003) *Public Health and Society*. Basingstoke: Palgrave Macmillan.

Cote, S. and Healy, T. (2001) *Indications of Public Health in the English Regions 7: Mental Health North East Public Health Observatory (NEPHO) and the National Mental Health Observatory (MHO)*. York: Association of Public Health Observatories (APHO).

Coughlin, S. S. (2006) 'Ethical issues in epidemiologic research and public health practice', *Emerging Themes in Epidemiology*, 3: 16.

Coulter, A. (2006) 'Patient engagement: why is it important?', in E. Andersson, J. Tritter and R. Wilson (eds), *Healthy Democracy: The Future of Involvement in Health and Social Care*. London: Involve/NCI.

Coyle, D. and Davies, L. (1996) 'How to Assess Cost-Effectiveness: Elements of a sound economic evaluation', in M. F. Drummond and A. Maynard (eds) *Purchasing and Providing Cost-Effective Health Care*. London: Churchill Livingstone. pp. 66–79.

Crisp, R. (1998) 'Ethics', in E. Craig (ed.), *Routledge Encyclopaedia of Philosophy*. London: Routledge.

Crombie, I. (1996) *The Pocket Guide to Critical Appraisal*. London: Sage.

Crone, D., Johnston, L. and Grant, T. (2004) 'Maintaining quality in exercise referral schemes: a case study of professional practice', *Primary Healthcare Research*, 5: 1–7

Cummins, S. and Macintyre, S. (2002) 'A systematic study of an urban foodscape: the price and availability of food in greater Glasgow', *Urban Studies*, 39: 2115-2130.

Curtis, S. (2004) *Health and Inequality*. London: Sage.

Dahlgren, G. and Whitehead, M. (1991) *Policies and Strategies to Promote Social Equity in Health*. Stockholm: Institute of Future Studies.

Dallongeville, J., Helbecque, N., Cottel, D., Amoulyel, P. and Meirhaeghe, A. (2003) 'The Gly16-Arg16 and Gln27-Glu27 polymorphisms of beta2-adrenergic receptor are associated with metabolic syndrome in men', *Journal of Clinical Endocrinol Metab*, 88: 4862-4866.

Darmon, N., Coupel, J., Deheeger, M. and Briend, A. (2002) 'Dietry inadequacies observed in homeless men visiting an emergency night shelter in Paris', *Public Health Nutrition*, 4: 155-161.

Davidoff, F., Haynes, B., Sackett, D. and Smith, R. (1995) 'Evidence based medicine', *British Medical Journal*, 310: 1085–6.

Davies, M. and Macdowall, W. (2006) *Health Promotion Theory*. Maidenhead Open University Press.

Davies, P. (1999) 'What is evidence based education?' *British Journal of Educational Studies*, 47(2): 108–21.

Davis, T. C. (1993) 'Rapid estimate of adult literacy in medicine: a shortened screening instrument', *Family Medicine*, 25: 391–5.

Davison, C., Davey Smith, G. and Frankel, S. (1991) 'Lay epidemiology and the prevention paradox: the implications of coronary candidacy for health education', *Sociology of Health and Illness*, 13(1): 1–19.

Dawson, K. A., Schneider, M. A., Fletcher, P. C. and Bryden, P. J. (2007) 'Examining gender differences in the health behaviours of Canadian university students', *J R Soc Health*, 127(1): 38–44.

DCMS/Strategy Unit (2002) *Game Plan: A Strategy for Delivering Government's Sport and Physical Activity Objectives*. London: Cabinet Office.

DeBell, D. (ed.) (2007) *Public Health Practice and the School Age Population*. London: Hodder Arnold.

Deeny, P. and McFetridge, B. (2005) 'The impact of disaster on culture, self and identity: increased awareness by healthcare professionals is needed', *Nursing Clinics of North America*, 40(3): 431–40.

Deeny, P., Davies, K., Gillespie, M. and Spencer, W. (2007) 'Global issues in disaster relief nursing', in T. G. Veenema (ed.), *Disaster Nursing and Emergency Preparedness for Chemical, Biological, and Radiological Terrorism and Other Hazards*. New York: Springer.

De Irala-Estevez, J., Groth, M. J. L., Olstersdorf, U., Prattala, R. and Martinez-Gonzalez, M. (2000) ' A systematic review of socioe-economic differences in food habits in Europe: consumption of fruit and vegetables', *European Journal of Clinical Nutrition*, 54: 706–14.

Department for Children, Schools and Families (DCSF) (2007a) *Care Matters: Transforming the Lives of Children and Young People in Care*. London: DfES.

Department for Children, Schools and Families (2007b) *The Children's Plan: Building Brighter Futures*. Retrieved 20 March 2008, from http://www.dfes.gov.uk/publications/ childrensplan/downloads/The_Childrens_Plan.pdf

Devaney, B., Schochet, P., Thornton, C., Fasciano, N. and Gavin, A. (1993) *Evaluating the Effects of School Health Interventions on School Performance: Design Report*. Princton, NJ: Mathematica Policy Reseach.

DfES (1999) *National Healthy Schools Standard Guidance*. Retrieved 20 March 2008, from http://www.wiredforhealth.gov.uk/PDF/Brochurenew.pdf

DfES (2003) *Every Child Matters: Next Step*. Retrieved 20 March 2008, from http://www.dfes.gov.uk/everychildmatters/pdfs/EveryChild

DfES (2005) *Common Assessment Framework for Children and Young People*. London: DfES.

DfES (2005) *Youth Matters Green Paper*. Retrieved 24 March 2008, from www.dfes.gov.uk/consultations/downloadableDocs/Youth%20mattters%20pdf.pdf

DfES (2007a) *Care Matters: Time for Change*. London: DfES.

DfES (2007b) *The Children's Plan: Building Brighter Future*. Retrieved 20 March 2008, from http://www.dfes.gov.uk/publications/childrensplan/downloads/The_ Childrens_Plan.pdf

Department of Communities and Local Government (DCLG) (1996) *The Housing Act 1996*. London: The Stationery Office.

Department of Education and Skills (2003) *Change for Children*. Retrieved 20 March 2008, from http://www.dfes.gov.uk/everychildmatters

DH (Department of Health) (1984) *The Public Health (Control of Disease) Act*. London: Department of Health.

DH (1987) *Promoting Better Health: Command No. 249*. London: Department of Health.

DH (1988) *Griffiths Report: Community Care: Agenda for Action (The Griffiths Community Care Report)*. London: HSMO.

The Public Health (Infectious Diseases) Regulations (1988).

DH (1992) *The Health of the Nation – A Strategy for Health in England*. London: HSM.

DH (1997) *The New NHS: Modern, Dependable*. London: Department of Health.

DH (1998a) *Our Healthier Nation*. London: The Stationery Office.

DH (1998b) *Tackling Drugs to Build a Better Britain: The Government's Ten Year Strategy for Tackling Drug Misuse*. London: Department of Health.

DH (1998c) *Making a Difference: Strengthening the Nursing, Midwifery and Health Visiting Contribution to Health and Healthcare*. Retrieved December 19 2007, from www.dh.gov.uk/prod_consum_dh/groups/dh_digitalassets/@dh/@en/documents/digitalasset/dh_4074704.pdf

DH (1999) *The National Service Framework for Mental Health: Modern Standards and Service Models*. London: Department of Health.

DH (2000a) *Access to Mainstream Health Promotion and Disease Prevention Programmes*. London: Department of Health.

DH (2000b) *The NHS Plan: A Plan for Investment, A Plan for Reform*. London: Department of Health.

DH (2000c) *Coronary Heart Disease: National Service Framework for Coronary Heart Disease: Modern Standards and Service Models*. London: Department of Health.

DH (2001a) *Exercise Referral Systems: A National Quality Assurance Framework*. London: Department of Health.

DH (2001b) *Making it Happen. A Guide to Delivering Mental Health Promotion*. London: Department of Health.

DH (2001c) *National Service Framework for Older People*. Retrieved 6 January 2008, from http://www.dh.gov.uk/en/Publicationsandstatistics/Publications/Publications PolicyAndGuidance/DH_4003066

DH (2001d) *The National Service Framework for Diabetes*. London: Department of Health.

DH (2001e) *UK Guidance on Best Practice in Vaccine Administration*. London: Shire Hall Communications.

DH (2002) *Getting Ahead of the Curve: A Strategy for Infectious Diseases*. London: Department of Health.

DH (2003a) *Taking a Public Health Approach in the Workplace*. London: Department of Health.

DH (2003b) *Chief Medical Office Letter: (PL/CMO/2003/1) Planned Hib Vaccination Catch-up Campaign*. London: Department of Health.

DH (2003c) *Fast-Forwarding Primary Care Mental Health 'Gateway' Workers*. London: Department of Health.

DH (2003d) *Liberating the Public Health Talents of Community Practitioners and Health Visitors*. London: Department of Health.

DH (2003e) *Mental Health Policy Implementation Guide: Support, Time and Recovery (STR) Workers*. London: Department of Health.

DH (2003f) *Tackling Health Inequalities: A Programme for Action*. London: Department of Health.

DH (2004a) *At Least Five a Week: Evidence on the Impact of Physical Activity and its Relationship to Health: A Report from the Chief Medical Officer*. London: The Stationery Office.

DH (2004b) *Choosing Health: Making Healthy Choices Easier*. London: Department of Health.

DH (2004c) *Health, Work and Wellbeing: A Strategy for the Health and Wellbeing of Working Age People*. London: Department of Health.

DH (2004d) *National Service Framework for Children, Young People and Maternity Services*. Retrieved 20 March 2008, from www.dh.gov.uk/en/Healthcare/National ServiceFrameworks/ChildrenServices

DH (2004e) *Taking a Public Health Approach in the Workplace*. London: Department of Health.

DH (2005a) *Commissioning a Patient-led NHS*. London: Department of Health.

DH (2005b) *Delivering Choosing Our Health: Making Healthier Choices Easier*. London: Department of Health.

DH (2005c) *Health Protection in the 21st Century: Understanding the Burden of Disease*. London: Department of Health.

DH (2005d) *National Healthy Schools Status: Guide for School*. Retrieved 20 January 2007, from http://www.wiredforhealth.gov.uk

DH (2006a) *The Local Government and Public Involvement in Health Act: Publications Legislation Section*. Retrieved 21 January 2008, from http://www.dh.gov.uk/en/ Publicationsandstatistics/Publications/PublicationsLegislation/DH_076445

DH (2006b) *The Expert Patients Programme*. London: Department of Health.

DH (2006c) *Chronic Obstructive Pulmonary Disease National Service Framework*. Retrieved 6 March, 2008, from www.dh.gov.uk/en/Healthcare/NationalService Frameworks/DH_4138532

DH (2006d) *Diabetes Commissioning Toolkit*. London: Department of Health.

DH (2006e) *Our Health, Our Care, Our Say: A New Direction for Community Services*. London: Department of Health.

DH (2006f) *Essence of Care Benchmarks for Promotion of Health*. London: Department of Health.

DH (2006g) *Transition: Getting it Right for Young People: Improving the Transition of Young People with Long Term Conditions from Children's to Adult Health Services*. London: Department of Health.

DH (2007a) *Consultation on Changing the Age of Sale for Tobacco: Report on Consultation*. London: Department of Health.

DH (2007b) *Partnerships for Better Health*. London: Department of Health.

DH (2007c) *Analysis of the National Childhood Obesity Database 2005–06*. Retrieved 10 December 2007, from http://www.dh.gov.uk/en/Publicationsandstatistics/ Publications/PublicationsStatistics/DH_063565

DH (2007d) *Commissioning Framework for Health and Wellbeing*. London: Department of Health.

DH (2007e) *Facing the Future: The Governments' Response*. London: Department of Health.

DH (2007f) *Review of Parts II, V and VI of the Public Health (Control of Disease) Act 1984: Report on Consultation* (Department of Health). Retrieved 21 June 2007, from http://www.dh.gov.uk/en/Consultations/Responsestoconsultations/DH_080384

DH (2007g) *World Class Commissioning*. London: Department of Health.

DH (2008a) *The Child Health Promotion Programme: Pregnancy and the First Five Years*. Retrieved 20 March 2008, from http://www.dh.gov.uk/en/Publicationsandstatistics/ Publications/DH_083645

key concepts in public health

DH (2008b) *Expanding the Psychological Therapies Workforce.* Retrieved 21 March 2008, from http://www.dh.gov.uk/en/News/Recentstories/DH_083176

DHSS (Department of Health and Social Security) (1942) *Beveridge Report – Social Insurance and Allied Services.* London: HSMO.

DHSS (1976) *Prevention and Health: Everybody's Business.* London: DHSS.

DHSS (1987) *Promoting Better Health.* London: HSMO.

DHSS (1988) *Community Care: Agenda for Action.* London: DHSS.

Department of Minerals and Energy (2003) *White Paper on the Renewable Energy Policy of the Republic of South Africa.* Pretoria: Department of Minerals and Energy.

Department of Minerals and Energy (1998) *White Paper on the Renewable Energy Policy of the Republic of South Africa.* Cape Town: Department of Minerals and Energy.

Dickersin, K. and Min, Y. I. (1993) 'Publication bias: the problem that won't go away', *Ann N Y Acad Sci,* 703: 135–46.

Di Gallo, A., Barton, J. and Parry-Jones, W. L. I. (1997) 'Road traffic accidents: early psychological consequences in children and adolescents', *British Journal of Psychiatry,* 170: 358–62.

Disability Discrimination Act (1996) *The Disability Discrimination Act: Analysis of Data from the ONS Omnibus Survey 1996–2006.*

Dolan, F. E. (1994) *Dangerous Familiars – Representation of Domestic Crime in England 1550–1700.* London: Cornell University Press

Donaldson, L. J. and Donaldson, R. J. (2003) *Essential Public Health.* London: Petroc Press.

Dowler, E. and Calvert, C. (1995) *Nutrition and Diet in Lone-parent Families in London.* London: Family Policy Study Centre for the Joseph Rowntree Foundation.

Drummond, M., Cooke, J. and Walley, T. (1997) 'Economic evaluation under managed competition: Evidence form the UK', *Social Science and Medicine,* 45(4): 583–95.

Dubois, L. and Girard, M. (2001) 'Social position and nutrition: A gradient relationship in Canada and the USA', *European Journal of Clinical Nutrition,* 55: 366–73.

Dugdill, L., Graham, R. and McNair, F. (2005) 'Exercise referral: the public health panacea for physical activity promotion? A critical perspective of exercise referral schemes; their development and evaluation', *Ergonoimics,* 48(11): 1390–410.

Dunstan, D. W., Zimmet, P. A. O., Slade, R., Harper, S. and Burke, L. (2003) *Diabetes and Physical Activity.* (International Diabetes Institute). Retrieved 26 November 2007, from http://www.dav.org.au/docs/pdfs/20041122115847.pdf

Earle, S. (2007) 'Promoting public health: exploring the issues', in S. Earle (ed.), *Theory and Research in Promoting Public Health.* London: Sage.

Earle, S., Lloyd, C. E., Sidell, M. and Spurr, S. (2007) *Theory and Research in Promoting Public Health.* London: Sage.

Earle, S., Sidell, M. and Spurr, S. (2007) *Theory and Research in Promoting Public Health.* London: Sage.

Easterling, D. V., Gallagher, K. M. and Lodwick, D. G. (2003) *Promoting Health at the Community Level.* London: Sage.

Eastern Region Public Health Observatory (ERPHO) (2002) *InphoRM 1: Introduction to Health Equity Audit.* Cambridge: ERPHO.

Eastern Region Public Health Observatory (ERPHO) (2006) *Briefing 14: Assessing, Measuring and Monitoring Local Health Inequalities.* Cambridge: ERPHO.

Ebrahim, S. (2005) 'Health of elderly people', in R. Detels, J. McEwen, R. Beaglehole and H. Tanaka (eds), *Oxford Textbook of Public Health*. Oxford: Oxford University Press.

Economic and Social Research Council (2004) *Participation and Democracy: A Health Check for British Democracy*. Swindon: ESRC Publications.

Efstathiou, A., Grant, D. and Maxwell, S. M. (2004) 'The ownership and use of small kitchen domestic appliances: case study, Liverpool', *International Journal of Consumer Studies*, 28(3): 305–11.

Ekman, I., Schaufelberger, M., Kjellgren, I., Swedberg, K. and Granger, B. (2007) 'Standard medication information is not enough: poor concordance of patient and nurse perceptions', *The Authors Journal Compilation*, 60(2): 181–6.

El Ansari, W. (2003) 'Educational partnerships for health: do stakeholders perceive similar outcomes?' *Journal of Public Health Management and Practice*, 9(2): 136–56.

El Ansari, W. and Phillips, C. J. (2001a) 'Empowering healthcare workers in Africa: partnerships in health – beyond the rhetoric towards a model', *Critical Public Health*, 11(3): 231–52.

El Ansari, W. and Phillips, C. J. (2001b) 'Interprofessional collaboration: a stakeholder approach to evaluation of voluntary participation in community partnerships', *Journal of Interprofessional Care*, 15(4): 351–68.

El Ansari, W. and Phillips, C. (2004) 'The costs and benefits of participants in community partnerships. A paradox?' *Health Promotion Practice*, 5(1): 35–48.

El Ansari, W., Phillips, C. J. and Hammick, M. (2001) 'Collaboration and partnerships: developing the evidence base', *Health and Social Care in the Community*, 9(4): 215–27.

El Ansari, W., Phillips, C. J. and Zwi, A. B. (2002) 'Narrowing the gap between academic professional wisdom and community lay knowledge: partnerships in South Africa', *Public Health*, 116(3): 151–9.

El Ansari, W., Phillips, C. J. and Zwi, A. B. (2004) 'Collaboration in health: public health nurses' perspectives', *Public Health Nursing*, 21(3): 278–87.

El Ansari, W., Maxwell, A., Stock, C., Mikolajczyk, R., Naydenova, V. and Krämer, A. (2007a) 'Nurse involvement in international research collaborations', *Nursing Standard*, 21(6): 35–40.

El Ansari, W., Maxwell, A. E., Mikolajczyk, R. T., Stock, C., Naydenova, V. and Krämer, A. (2007b) 'Promoting public health: benefits and challenges of a European wide research consortium on student health', *Central European Journal for Public Health*, 15(2): 58–65.

Ellis, R. and Hogard, E. (2006) 'The Trident: a three pronged method for evaluating clinical, social and educational innovations', *Evaluation*, 12(3): 372–83.

Endacott, R. (1997) 'Clarifying the concept of need: a comparison of two approaches to concept analysis', *Journal of Advanced Nursing*, 25: 471–76.

Engelke, M. and Engelke, S. (1992) 'Predictors of the home environment of high-risk infants', *Journal of Community Health Nursing*, 91(3): 171–18.

Enthoven, A. (1985) *Reflections on the Management of the NHS*. Oxford: Nuffield Provincial Hospital Trusts.

Ewles, L. and Simnett, I. (2003) *Promoting Health: A Practical Guide*. London: Bailliere Tindall.

Eyler, A., Baker, E., Cromer, L., King, A. and Brown, D. (1997) 'Physical activity and minority women: a qualitative approach', *Health Education and Behaviour*, 25: 640–52.

Falk-Rafael, A. (2005) 'Speaking truth to power: nursing's legacy and moral imperative', *Advances in Nursing Science*, 28(3): 212–23.

Fendrick, A., Javitt, J. C. and Chiang, Y. P. (1992) 'Cost-effectiveness of the screening and treatment of diabetic retinopathy', *International Journal of Technology Assessment in Healthcare*, 8(4): 694–707.

Fernando, S. (2003) 'Culture and ethnicity', in B. Hannigan and M. Coffey (eds), *The Handbook of Community Mental Health Nursing*. London: Routledge.

Ferner, R. E. (2003) 'Is concordance the primrose path to health?' Editorial in *British Medical Journal*, 327: 821–2.

Field, J. (2003) *Social Capital*. London: Routledge.

Field, J. (2008) *Social Capital*, 2nd edn. London: Routledge.

Firth, S. (2005) *Staying in or Standing Out*. London: Sage.

Fitzpatrick, M. (2001) *The Tyranny of Health: Doctors and the Regulation of Lifestyle*. London:

Fitzpatrick, M. (2004) 'From "nanny state" to "therapeutic state"', *British Journal of General Practice*, 54(505): 645.

Flaskerud, J. and Winsow, B. (1998) 'Conceptualizing vulnerable populations: health based research', *Nursing Research*, 47: 69–77.

Fleming, P. (2007) 'Public health: social context and action', in A. Scriven and S. Garmen (eds), *Public Health*. London: McGraw-Hill.

Fleming, P., Blair, P., Bacon, C., Bensley, D., Smith, I., Taylor, E., et al. (1996) 'Environment of infants during sleep and risk of the sudden infant death syndrome: results of 1993–1995 case-control study for confidential inquiry into stillbirths and deaths in infancy', *British Medical Journal*, 313(7051): 191–5.

Food Standards Agency (2002) *COT (Non-food) Statement on the Study by the Small Area Health Statistics Unit (SAHSU) on Health Outcomes in Populations Living Around Landfill Sites*. Retrieved 8 August 2007, from http://www.food.gov.uk/science/ouradvisors/toxicity/statements/cotstatements2002/sahsulandfill

Foucault, M. (ed.) (1991) *Governmentality*. Hemel Hempstead: Harvester Wheatsheaf.

French, J. and Blair-Stevens, C. (2006) *It's Our Health! Realising the Potential of Social Marketing*. London: National Consumer Council of Social Marketing.

Friis, R. H. and Sellers, T. A. (2004) *Epidemiology for Public Health Practice*, 3rd edn. Boston: Jones and Bartlett.

Fry, H., Ketteridge, S. and Marshall, S. (2000) *A Handbook for Teaching and Learning in Higher Education*. London: Kogan Page.

Galazka, A. (1993) *The Immunological Basis for Immunization. Module 1: General Immunology*. Geneva: World Health Organization.

Garmen, S. (2007) *Public Health: Social Context and Action*. London: McGraw-Hill.

Gibney, M. J. and Nutrition Society (2004) *Public Health Nutrition*. Oxford: Blackwell Science.

Gibson, A. (ed.) (2007) 'Does social capital have a role to play in the health of communities?' in Douglas et al. (eds), *A Reader in Promoting Public Health – Challenge and Controversy*. London: Sage.

Giddens, A. (1991) *Modernity and Self-Identity: Self and Society in the Late Modern Age*. Stanford: Stanford University Press.

Gill, T. (2005) 'If you go down to the woods today: even today's current breed of battery-reared, celebrity-fed, techno-kids would, given the chance, rather be outside than stuck indoors surfing the net. Isn't it time we had the courage to let them go?', *Ecologist*, 35(8): 62–9.

Giskes, K., Turrell, G., Patterson, C. and Newman, B. (2002) 'Socio-economic differences in fruit and vegetable consumption among Australian adolescents and adults', *Public Health Nutrition*, 5: 663–9.

Goede, H. and El Ansari, W. (2003) *Partnership Work: the Health Service-Community Interface for the Prevention, Care and Treatment of HIV/AIDS Report of a WHO Consultation 5–6 December 2002*. Geneva: World Health Organization.

Goffman, E. (1961) *Stigma – Notes on the Management of Spoiled Identity*. New Jersey: Prentice Hall.

Goldenburg, M. J. (2005) 'Evidence-based ethics? On evidence-based practice and the "empirical turn" from normative ethics', *Medical Ethics*, 6: 11.

Goodman, E., Hinden, B. and Khandelwal, S. (2000) 'Accuracy of teen and parental reports of obesity and body mass index', *Paediatrics*, 106: 52–8.

Goodman, J. (2002) *Moral panic: HIV and AIDS*. Retrieved 28 June 2007, from http://www.joelgoodman.co.uk/files/pdfs/moralpanic.pdf

Gordis, L. (2005) *Epidemiology*. Philadelphia: Elsevier.

Gordon, D. et al. (eds) (1999) *Inequalities in Health: The Evidence*. Bristol: Policy Press.

Gordon, M. (2002) 'Illiteracy in rheumatoid arthritis patients as determined by the rapid estimate of adult literacy in medicine (REALM) score', *Rheumatology*, 41: 750–4.

Gorsky, M. (2007) 'Local leadership in public health: the role of the medical officer of health in Britain, 1872–1974', *Journal of Epidemiology and Community Health*, 61: 468–72.

Gostin, L. O. (2000) *Public Health Law: Power, Duty and Restraint*. New York: University of California Press.

Gostin, L. O. (2002) *Public Health Law and Ethics: A Reader*. New York: University of California Press.

Graham, H. (1993) *Hardship and Health in Women's Lives in Hemel Hempstead*. London: Harvester Wheatsheaf.

Graham, H. and Kelly, M. (2004) *Health Inequalities: Concepts, Frameworks and Policy*. London: Health Development Agency.

Gray, M. (2004) 'Evidence-based policy making', *British Medical Journal*, 329: 988–9.

Green, L. and Kreuter, M. (1999) *Health Promotion Planning: An Educational and Environmental Approach*, 3rd edn. Mountain View, CA: Mayfield.

Greenhalgh, T. (2006) *How to Read a Paper: Getting your Bearings*, 3rd edn. London: British Medical Journal.

Griffin, J., Arif, S. and Mufti, A. (2003) *Immunology and Haematology*. London: Mosby.

Griffiths, S. and Hunter, D. (2007) *New Perspectives in Public Health*, 2nd edn. Oxford: Radcliffe.

Grundy, E. (2004) *Demography and Public Health*. Oxford: Oxford University Press.

Guardian (2007a) *Smoking Ban Brings Big Cut in Heart Attacks in Scotland, Study Finds*. Retrieved 8 March 2008, from http://www.guardian.co.uk/uk/2007/sep/11/health.smoking

Guardian (2007b) 'Knowing what is best' (Leader), *The Guardian*, 3 July.

Guyatt, G. and Rennie, D. (2002) *Users' Guide to the Medical Literature: A Manual for Evidence-based Clinical Practice*. Chicago: AMA Press.

Hall, D. and Elliman, D. (2006) *Health for all Children*. Oxford: University of Oxford Press.

Hallfors, D., Cho, H., Livert, D. and Kadushin, C. (2002) 'Fighting back against substance abuse: are community coalitions winning?' *American Journal of Preventive Medicine*, 23(4): 237–45.

Hammond, J., Brodie, D. and Bundred, P. (1997) 'Exercise on prescription: guidelines for health professionals', *Health Promotion International*, 12(1): 33–41.

Hancock, H. and Campbell, S. (2006) 'Impact of the Leading an Empowered Organisation Programme', *Nursing Standards*, 20(19): 41–8.

Harland, J., White, M., Drinkwater, C., Chinn, D., Farr, L. and Howel, D. (1999) 'The Newcastle exercise project: a randomised controlled trial of methods to promote physical activity in primary care', *British Medical Journal*, 319: 828–32.

Harris, J. (1998) Manchester: Centre for Social Ethics and Policy, University of Manchester as cited in NHS London Health Observatory *Briefing on Water Fluoridation for London SHA and PCT CEs and DsPH*. Retrieved June 13 2007, from www.lho.org.uk/HIL/Determinants_Of_Health/Environment/Fluoridation.aspx#reports

Harris, J. (2005) *Double Trouble: Combining Research and Development. 11th International Conference on Qualitative Evidence in Health Care*. Uttrech, Holland.

Harrison, L. (1999) *Student Mental Health*. Retrieved 14 November 2007, from http/:www.brookes.ac.uk

Harrison, S. and Mort, M. (1998) 'Which champions, which people? public and user involvement in healthcare as a technology of legitimation', *Social Policy and Administration*, 32(1): 60–70.

Harrison, S., Dowswell, G. and Milewa, T. (2002) 'Public and user "involvement" in the UK National Health Service', *Health and Social Care in the Community*, 10(2): 63–6.

Hasler, F. (2006) 'Partners in participation? Involving people who use social care services', in E. Andersson, J. Tritter and R. Wilson (eds), *Healthy Democracy: The Future of Involvement in Health and Social Care*. London: Involve/NCI.

Hastings, G. (2007) *Social Marketing: The Potential*. London: Butterworth-Heinenmann.

Hawtin, M., Hughes, G. and Percy-Smith, J. (1999) *Community Profiling: Auditing Social Needs*. Buckingham: Open University Press.

Health Communication Unit (2007) *Health Communication*. Retrieved 20 March 2008, from http://www.thcu.ca/infoandresources/health_communication.htm

Health Protection Agency Act 2004 424, c41-71 Cong. Rec. pp.1-88 (2004).

Health Protection Agency (2007) *Chemical Hazards and Poison Division*. Retrieved 31 July 2007, from http://hpa.org.uk/chemicals/default.htm

Health and Safety at Work etc Act (HSWA) 1974, Health and Safety Executive SI 1974/1439 (1974).

Health and Safety Executive (2004) *Worker Involvement in Health and Safety Management*. HSE: London.

Health and Safety Executive (2004a). *Managing Absence in the Public Sector*. London: Health and Safety Executive

Health and Safety Executive (2007) *Health and Safety Statistics 2006/2007*. HSE: London.

Health and Social Care Bill (2007) *Health and Social Care Bill*. Retrieved June 12 2008, from www.commonsleader.gov.uk/output/page2030.asp#

Hearns, A. and Deeny, P. (2007) 'The value of support for aid workers in complex emergencies: a phenomenological study', *Disaster Management and Response*, 5(2): 28–35.

Helbert, M. (2006) *Flesh and Bones of Immunology*. London: Mosby.

Henderson, L., Gregory, J. and Swan, G. (2002) *The National Diet and Nutrition Survey: Adults Ages 19 to 64 Years. Volume 1 Types and Quantities of Foods Consumed*. London: The Stationery Office.

Hewitt, M. and Percy-Smith, J. (2007) *Community Profiling: A Practical Guide*, 2nd edn. Buckingham: Open University Press.

Hill, A. and Spittlehouse, C. (2003) *What is Critical Appraisal?* Vol 3, number 2. Hayward Medical Communications. from www.evidence-based-medicine.co.uk

Hillsdon, M., Foster, C., Naidoo, B. and Crombie, H. (2004) *The Effectiveness of Public Health Interventions for Increasing Physical Activity among Adults: A Review of Reviews*. London: Department of Health.

Hivert, M. F., Langlois, M. F., Bérard, P., Cuerrier, J. P. and Carpentier, A. C. (2007) 'Prevention of weight gain in young adults through a seminar-based intervention program', *International Journal of Obesity*, 31(8): 1262–9.

HM Treasury (2002) *Securing our Future: Taking a Long-term View*. London: HM Treasury.

HM Treasury (2004) *Securing Good Health for the Whole Population*. London: HM Treasury.

Holland, W. W., Stewart, S. and Masseria, C. (2006) *Policy Brief: Screening in Europe*. Retrieved 13 December 2007, from http://www.euro.who.int/Document/E88698.pdf

Holroyd, G. (2002) 'Partnerships and collaborations: the promise of participation', in L. Jones, M. Sidell and J. Douglas (eds), *The Challenge of Promoting Health: Exploration and Action*. Basingstoke: Macmillan/Open University.

Home Office (2005) *Domestic Violence: A National Report*. London: Home Office.

Hooper, J. and Longworth, P. (2002) *Health Needs Assessment Workbook*. London: Health Development Agency.

Horne, R. (2006) 'Compliance, adherence and concordance: implications for asthma treatment', *Chest*, 130(1): 65–72.

The Human Rights Act 1998, Home Office (1998).

Hunter, D. J. (2003) *Public Health Policy*. Cambridge: Polity Press.

IFRC (International Federation of Red Cross and Red Crescent Societies) (2001) *World Disasters Report 2001: Focus on Recovery*. Geneva: IFRC.

IFRC (2005) *World Disasters Report 2005: Focus on Information*. Geneva: IFRC.

Illich, I. (1976) *Limits to Medicine: Medical Nemesis: the Expropriation of Health*. London: Marion Boyars.

Institute for Volunteering Research (2004) *Volunteering for All: Exploring the Link between Volunteering and Social Exclusion*. London: Institute for Volunteering Research.

Involve (2005) *People and Participation: How to Put Citizens at the Heart of Decision-making*. London: Involve.

Jackson, S. F., Cleverly, S., Poland, B., Robertson, A., Burman, D., Goodstadt, M. and Salsberg, L. (1997) *Half Full or Half Empty? Concepts and Research Design for a Study of Community Capacity*. Ontario: City of North York Public Health Department Publishing.

Janeway, C., Travers, P., Walport, M. and Shlomik, M. (2005) *Immunobiology*. London: Churchill Livingstone.

Jeffery, J. (2006) 'Governance for a sustainable future', *Journal of the Royal Institute of Public Health*, 120: 604–8.

Jenkins, S. (2007) 'Nest the anti-smoking Guardianistas will be coming for dogs and cats', *The Guardian*, 16 July.

Jones, A. (2008) *Applied Econometrics for Health Economists*, 2nd edn. London: Office of Health Economics.

JRF (Joseph Rowntree Foundation) (2005) *The Older People's Inquiry: 'That Little Bit of Elp'*. Retrieved 16 December 2007, from http://www.jrf.org.uk/bookshop/ebooks/briefing03.pdf

Kals, E. and Montada, L. (1999) 'Emotional affinity toward nature as a motivational basis to protect nature', *Environment and Behaviour*, 31(2): 178–202.

Kassianos, G. (2001) *Immunization: Childhood and Travel Health*. Oxford: Blackwell Science.

Katz, J. (1997) *The Digital Citizen Survey*. Conducted by the Luntz Research Company for Wired magazine and the Merrill Lynch Forum.

Katz, J., Peberdy, A. and Douglas, J. (2000) *Promoting Health Knowledge and Practice*. London: The Open University.

Katz, E. and Lazarsfeld, P. (1955) 'Personal influence: the part played by people in the flow of mass communication', in K. Tones and J. Green (eds), *Health Promotion Planning and Strategies*. London: Sage.

Kelly, A. and Symonds, A. (2003) *The Social Construction of Community Nursing*. Basingstoke: Macmillan.

Kendall, L. (2007) 'Second thoughts: healthcare is failing those who most need it', *The Guardian*, 28 November.

Kendrick, T., Simons, L., Mynors-Wallis, L., Gray, A., Lathlean, J., Pickering, R. et al. (2006) 'Cost-effectiveness of referral for generic care or problem-solving treatment from community mental health nurses, compared with usual general practitioner care for common mental disorders Randomised controlled trial', *British Journal of Psychiatry*, 18(9): 50–59.

Kennedy, A., Reeves, D., Bower, B., Lee, V., Middleton, E., Richardson, G. et al. (2007) 'The effectiveness and cost effectiveness of a national lay-led self care support programme for patients with long-term conditions: a pragmatic randomised controlled trial', *Journal of Epidemiology and Community Health*, 61: 254–61.

Kennedy, B. P., Kawachi, I., Glass, R. and Prothrow-Stith, D. (1998) 'Income distribution, socioeconomic status and self-rated health in the United States: multilevel analysis', British Medical Journal, 317: 917–21.

Kennedy, E. T., Bowman, S. A. and Powell, R. (1999) 'Dietary-fat intake in the US population', *Journal of the American College of Nutrition*, 18(3): 207–12.

Kennedy, I. (2001) *Learning from Bristol: The Report of the Public Inquiry into Children's Heart Surgery at the Bristol*. London: HMSO.

Kennedy, L. and Ling, M. (eds) (1997) *Nutrition Education for Low-income Groups – Is There a Role?* Berlin: WZB.

Kibble, A. J. and Saunders, P. (2001) 'The public health significance of contaminated land', in R. Hestor and R. Harrison (eds), *Environmental Science and Technology, No. 16: Contaminated Land*. London: The Royal Society of Chemistry.

Kickbusch, I. (2001) 'Health literacy: addressing the health and education divide', *Health Promotion International*, 16(3): 289–97.

King, W. D., Darlington, G. and Kreiger, N. (1993) 'Response of a cancer registry to reports of disease clusters', *British Journal of Cancer*, 29: 1418–25.

King's Fund (2004a). *Public Attitudes to Public Health Policy*. London: King's Fund.

King's Fund (2004b) *Leadership at the Point of Care*. Retrieved 28 March 2008, from http://www.kingsfund.org.uk/current_projects/point_of_care/index.html

Kinzie, W. R. (2005) 'Instructional design strategies for health behaviour change', *Patient Education Council*, 56: 3–15.

Kitzman, H., Olds, D., Sidora, K., Henderson, C., Hanks, C. and Cole, R. (2000) 'Enduring effects of nurse home visitation on maternal life course: a 3 year follow up of a randomised trial', *Journal of the American Medical Association*, 283(15): 1983–9.

Kohler, L. (1998) 'Child public health: a new basis for child health workers', *European Journal of Public Health*, 8: 253–5.

Kotler, P. and Lee, N. (2006) *Marketing in the Public Sector: A Roadmap for Improved Performance*. London: Financial Times/ Prentice-Hall.

Kotler, P. and Zaltman, G. (1971) 'Social marketing: an approach to planned social change', *Journal of Marketing*, 35: 3–12.

Kotler, P., Roberto, N. and Lee, N. (2002) *Social Marketing. Improving the Quality of Life*. California: Sage.

Kralik, D., Price, K., Warren, J. and Koch, T. (2006) 'Issues in data generation using e-mail group conversations for nursing research', *Journal of Advances Nursing*, 53(2): 213–20.

Krieger, N. (2001) 'Theories for social epidemiology in the 21st century: an ecosocial perspective', *International Journal of Epidemiology*, 30(4): 668–77.

Kunkel, D., Wilcox, B. L., Cantor, J., Palmer, E., Linn, S. and Dowrick, P. (2004) *Report of the APA Task Force on Advertising and Children*. Retrieved 18 March 2007, from http://www.apa.org/releases/childrenads.pdf

Labonte, R. and Robertson, A. (1996) 'Delivering the goods, showing our stuff: the case for a constructivist paradigm for health promotion research and practice', *Health Education Quarterly*, 23: 431–47.

Labour Research Department (2004) *An Overview of the Services and Activities of the Labour Research Department*. Retrieved 23 March 2007, from http://www.tssa.org.uk/article-1.php3?id_article-2118

Lachance, L. L., Houle, C. R., Cassidy, E. F., Bourcier, E., Cohn, J. H. and Orians, C. E. (2006) 'Collaborative design and implementation of a multisite community coalition evaluation', *Health Promotion Practice*, 7(2): 44S–55S.

Lalonde, M. (1974) *A New Perspective on the Health of Canadians*. Ottawa: Information Canada.

Last, J. M. (2007) *A Dictionary of Public Health*. Oxford: Oxford University Press.

Last, J. M. (ed.) (2007) *A Dictionary of Public Health*. New York: Oxford University Press.

Laverack, G. (2005) *Public Health: Power, Empowerment and Professional Practice*. Basingstoke: Macmillan.

Layard, R. (2005) *Happiness – Lessons from a New Science*. London: Penguin.

Leavell, H. and Clarke, E. G. (1965) *Preventative Medicine for the Doctor and his Community*. New York: McGraw-Hill.

Lee, B. A., Price-Spratlen, T. and Kanan, J. W. (2003) 'Determinants of homelessness in metropolitan areas', *Journal of Urban Affairs*, 25(3): 335–56.

Lenihan, P. (2005) 'MAPP and the evolution of planning in public health practice', *Journal of Public Health Management Practice*, 11(5): 381–6.

Looker, K. J. and Hallett, T. B. (2006) 'Individual freedom versus collective responsibility: too many rights make a wrong?' 4, *Emerging Themes in Epidemiology*, 3: 14–17.

Louv, R. (2005) *Last Child in the Woods: Saving our Children from Nature-deficit Disorder*. New York: Workman.

Luck, M., Bamford, M. and Williamson, P. (2000) *Men's Health – Perspectives, Diversity and Paradox*. Oxford: Blackwell Science.

Lunt, J. and Coyle, D. (2007) *Person Centred Thinking Minibook for People who Use Mental Health Services*. Stockport: The Learning Community for Person Centred Practices.

Lupton, D. (1995) *The Imperative of Health: Public health and the regulated body*. London: Sage.

MacDonald, M. A. (2004) 'From miasma to fractals: the epidemiology revolution and public health nursing', *Public Health Nursing*, 21(4): 380–91.

Mackereth, C. (2007) *Community Development: New Challenges, New Opportunities*. London: CPHVA.

MacRae, G., Regehr, M., McKenzie, H. and Henteleff, M. (2004) 'Teaching practicing surgeons critical appraisal skills with an Internet-based journal club: a randomized, controlled trial', *Surgery*, 136(3): 641–6.

Making Ends Meet: A website for managing the money in social services (n.d.) Social Services Inspectorate & Audit Commission. Retrieved 22 August 2007, from http://www.joint-reviews.gov.uk/money/Commissioning/2-contents.html

March, D. and Susser, E. (2006) 'The eco- in eco epidemiology', *International Journal of Epidemiology*, 35(6): 1379–83.

Marchette, C., Meyer, P. S. and Ausubel, J. H. (2007) 'Human population dynamics revisited with the logistic model: how much can be modeled and predicted?' *Technological Forecasting and Social Change*, 52: 1–30.

Marmot, M., Banks, J., Blundell, R., Lessof, C. and Nazroo, J. (2002) *Health, Wealth and Lifestyles of the Older Population in England: The 2002 English Longitudinal Study of Ageing*. London: Institute for Fiscal Studies.

Marmot, M. (2003) 'Self-esteem and health', *British Medical Journal*, 327: 574–5.

Marmot, M. and Wilkinson, R. (2001) 'Psychosocial and material pathways in the relation between income and health', *British Medical Journal*, 322: 1233–6.

Martin, C. J. and McQueen, D. V. (1989) *Readings for a New Public Health*. Edinburgh: Edinburgh University Press.

Masika, R. and Joekes, S. (1997) *Environmentally Sustainable Development and Poverty: A Gender Analysis Report prepared for the Gender Equality Unit*. Brighton: Swedish International Development Cooperation Agency.

Mason, T., Carlisle, C., Walkins, C. and Whitehead, E. (2001) *Stigma and Social Exclusion in Healthcare*. London: Routledge.

McDonald, G. (2006) *What is Mental Health in Mental Health Promotion across the Lifespan?* Milton Keynes: Open University Press.

McDonald, G. and O'Hara, K. (1998) *Ten Elements of Mental Health, its Promotion and Demotion: Implications for Practice*. Society of Health Education and Health Promotion Specialists.

McKeown, F. (2007) 'The experiences of older people on discharge from hospital following assessment by the public health nurse', *Journal of Clinical Nursing*, 16: 469–76.

McKeown, T. (1976) *The Role of Medicine: Dream, Mirage, or Nemesis?* London: Nuffield Provincial Hospitals Trust.

Medical Research Council (2002) *Working Group Report. Water Fluoridation and Health*. London: Medical Research Council.

Memon, A. (2006) 'Epidemiological understanding: an overview of basic concepts and study designs', in D. Pencheon, C. Guest, J. A. Melzer and M. Gray (eds), *Oxford Handbook of Public Health Practice*. Oxford: Oxford University Press.

Mental Health Foundation (2005) *GPs Should be Offering Exercise on Prescription to all Patients with Depression, Says New Report by the Mental Health Foundation*. Retrieved June 22 2008, from www.mentalhealth.org.uk/media/news-releases/news-releases-2005/29-march-2005/

The Mental Health Foundation (2005) *Up and Running: Exercise Therapy and the Treatment for Mild or Moderate Depression in Primary Care*. London: The Mental Health Foundation.

Menzies, D., Nair, A., Williamson, P. A., Schembri, S., Al-Khairalla, M. Z. H., Barnes, M. et al. (2006) 'Respiratory symptoms, pulmonary function, and markers of inflammation among bar workers before and after a legislative ban on smoking in public places', *JAMA*, 296: 1742–8.

Metcalfe, R. (2005) 'Compliance, adherence, concordance – what's in a NAME?' *Practical Neurology*, 5: 192–119.

Mikolajczyk , R. T., Maxwell, A. E., El Ansari, W., Naydenova, V., Stock, C., Ilieva, S. et al. (2007) 'Prevalence of depressive symptoms in university students from Germany, Denmark, Poland and Bulgaria', *Social Psychiatry and Psychiatric Epidemiology*, 43(2): 105–12.

Miller, A. B. and Vivek, G. (2004) *Screening*, 4th edn. Oxford: Oxford University Press.

Miller, W. R. and Rollnick, S. (2002) *Motivational Interviewing: Preparing People for Change*, 2nd edn. New York: Guildford.

Mind (2007) *Ecotherapy: The Green Agenda for Mental Health*. London: Mind.

Minkler, M. (1997) *Community Organization and Community Building for Health*. New Brunswick, NJ: Rutgers University Press.

Montessori, M. (1976) *From Childhood to Adolescence*. New York: Schocken.

Mooney, G. (2003) *Economics, Medicine and Health Care*. Harlow: Pearson Education.

Moore, T. and Lakha, R. (2006) *Tolley's Handbook of Disaster and Emergency Management: Principles and Practice*, 3rd edn. Oxford: Butterworth-Heinemann.

Morris, L. S. and Schulz, R. M. (1992) 'Patient compliance: an overview', *Journal of Clinical Pharmacology Therapy*, 17: 283–95.

MUCPP (Mangaung-University of the Orange Free State Community Partnership Programme) (1995) *Health For All: Building our Nation Together*. Bloemfontein, South Africa: MUCPP.

Muir Gray, J. A. (2001) *Evidence-based Healthcare: How to Make Health Policy and Management Decisions*. London: Churchill Livingstone.

Mulcahy, H. (2004) 'Vulnerable family as understood by public health nurses', *Community Practitioner*, 77: 257–60.

Myers, L. B. and Midence, L. (1998) *Adherence to Treatment in Medical Conditions*. New York, NJ: Harwood Academic.

Naidoo, J. and Wills, J. (2000) *Health Promotion Foundation for Practice*. Edinburgh: Harcourt.

Naidoo, J. and Wills, J. (2005) *Public Health and Health Promotion*. London: Baillière, Tindall.

Nardi, D. A. and Petr, M. P. J. (2003) *Community Health and Wellness Needs Assessment: A Step-by-step Guide*. New York: Thomson/Delmar Learning.

National Audit Office (2004) *Getting Citizens Involved: Community Participation in Neighbourhood Renewal*. London: National Audit Office.

Natural England (2008) *Natural England Works for People, Places and Nature to Conserve and Enhance Biodiversity, Landscapes and Wildlife in Rural, Coastal and Marine Areas*. Retrieved 3 April 2008, from http://www.naturalengland.org.uk

Navarro, V. (1976) *Medicine under Capitalism*. New York: Prodist.

NCCSDO (National Co-ordinating Centre for NHS Service Delivery and Organisation R & D) (2005) *Concordance, Adherence and Compliance in Medicine Taking*. London: NCCSDO.

Neiner, J., Howze, E. and Greaney, M. (2004) 'Using scenario planning in public health: anticipating alternative futures', *Health Promotion Practice*, 5(1): 69–79.

Nelson, T. F., Gortmaker, S. L., Subramanian, S. V. and Wechsler, H. (2007) 'Vigorous physical activity among college students in the United States', *Journal of Physical Activities Health*, 4(4): 495–508.

NESS (National Evaluation of Sure Start) (2005) *Research Report: Early Impacts of Sure Start Local Programmes on Children and Families*. Retrieved 20 August 2007, from http://www.ness.bbk.ac.uk/documents/activities/impact/1183.pdf

Newland, R. and Cowley, S. (2003) 'Investigating how health visitors define vulnerability', *Community Practitioner*, 76, 464–7.

NHS Insitute for Innovation and Improvement (2001) Leadership Qualities Framework. Retrieved 28 March 2008, from http://www.nhsleadershipqualities. nhs.uk/

NHS Institute for Innovation and Improvement (2005) *Improvement Leaders Guides*. Retrieved 28 March 2007, from www.institute.nhs.uk/building_capability/building_ improvement_capability/improvement_leaders%27_guides%3a_introduction.html

NHS Leadership Centre (2001) *NHS Leadership Qualities Framework*. Retrieved June 21 2008, from www.nhsleadershipqualities.nhs.uk/Portals/0/Technical_Research_ Paper_Summary.pdf

NHS Leadership Centre (2004) *Leadership Qualities Framework: A Good Practice Guide NHS Modernisation Agency*. London: NHS.

NICE (National Institute Clinical Excellence) (2006) *Cardiovascular Disease – Statins: Guidance*. London: NICE.

NICE (National Institute for Clinical Excellence) (2005) *Health Needs Assessment: A Practical Guide*. London: NICE.

NSHP (National Healthy School Programme) (2004) *Final Evaluation Report*. London: Department of Health.

Nicolau, B., Thompson, W. J., Steele, G. and Allison, P. J. (2007) 'Life-course epidemiology: concepts and theoretical models and its relevance to chronic oral conditions', *Community Dentistry and Oral Epidemiology*, 35(4): 241–9.

NSMC (National Social Marketing Centre) (2006) *It's Our Health*. London: NSMC.

NSMC (2007) *Social Marketing Big Pocket Guide*. London: NSMC.

NSO (National Statistics Online) (2004) Older people – population. Retrieved 7 November 2007, from http://www.statistics.gov.uk/CCI/nugget.asp?ID=874&Pos =3&ColRank=2&Rank=1000

Nursing and Midwifery Council (NMC) (2004) *Specialist Community Public Health Nursing*. Retrieved June 21 2008, from www.nmc-uk.org/aArticle.aspx?Article ID=2137

Nutbeam, D. (1996) 'Achieving best practice in health promotion: improving the fit between research and practice', *Health Education Research*, 11(3): 317–26.

Nutbeam, D. (1998) 'Health promotion glossary', *Health Promotion International*, 13: 349–64.

Nutbeam, D. (2000) 'Health literacy as a public health goal: a challenge for contemporary health education and communication strategies into the 21st century', *Health Promotion International*, 15(3): 259–67.

Nutrition Society (2007) *Voluntary Register of Nutritionists: Guide to Registration as a Nutritionist*. Cambridge: Nutrition Society.

NWPHO (North West Public Health Observatory) (2002) *Older People and Health in the North-west of England*. Retrieved 12 November 2007, from http://www.nwph. net/nwpho/Publications/olderp.pdf

Oakley, K. (2002) *Occupational Health Nursing*. London: Whurr.

Oakley, S. (2002) 'Design and analysis of social intervention studies in health', in A. Bowling and S. Ebrahim (eds), *Handbook of Health Research Methods*. Maidenhead: Open University Press.

O'Connor, E. M. (2001) 'Student mental health: secondary education no more', *Monitor on Psychology*, 32(8):

O'Donnell M. P. (2002) *Health Promotion in the Workplace*, 3rd edn. Toronto: Delmar Thomson Learning.

ODPM (Office for Deputy Prime Minister) (2005) *Creating Healthier Communities: A Resource Pack for Local Partnerships. Office for Public Sector Information Disability Discrimination Act (1995)*. London: HMSO.

OECD (2007) *Policy Coherence for Development Migration and Developing Countries*. Paris: OECD.

Office for National Statistics (2003) *Deaths by Age, Sex and Underlying Cause in England and Wales*. London: Stationery Office.

Office for National Statistics (2006) *Population Trends*. London: Office for National Statistics.

Ofsted (2001) *A Review of Evidence of the Impact on Schools of the Implementation of the National Healthy School Standard drawn from the Ofsted Database of Schools in England Inspected September 2000–July 2001*. London: Ofsted.

Oliver, M. (1996) *Understanding Disability from Theory to Practice*. London: Macmillan.

O'Neill, M. and Pederson, A. (1992) 'Building a methods bridge between policy analysis and healthy public policy', *Canadian Journal of Public Health*, 83: 25–30.

Orme, J., Powell, J., Taylor, P. and Grey, M. (2007) *Public Health for the 21st Century*. Maidenhead: McGraw-Hill/ Open University Press.

Osbourne, H. (2005) *Health Literacy from A-Z: Practical Ways to Communicate your Health Message*. London: Jones and Bartlett.

Oxfam (2007) *Weather Alert to Climate Alarm*. (Oxford Briefing paper). Oxford: Oxfam.

Patton, G. C., Carlin, J. B., Coffey, C., Wolfe, R., Hibbert, M. and Bowes, G. (1998) 'Depression, anxiety, and smoking initiation: a prospective study over 3 years', *Am J Public Health Nations Health*, 88(10): 518–22.

Payne, J. and Schulte, S. (2003) 'Mass media, public health, and achieving health literacy', *Journal of Health Communication*, 8: 124–5.

Pearce, N. (1996) 'Traditional epidemiology, modern epidemiology, and public health', *American Journal of Public Health*, 86(5): 678–82.

Pencheon, D., Melzer, D., Gray, M. and Guest, C. (2006) *Oxford Handbook of Public Health Practice*. New York: Oxford University Press.

Pilgrim, D. and Rogers, A. (2003) *Sociology of Mental Illness*, 3rd edn. Milton Keynes: Open University Press.

Pleasant, A. and Kuruvilla, S. (2008) 'A tale of two health literacies: public health and clinical approaches to health literacy', *Health Promotion International Advance*, 23(2): 152–9.

Plotkin, S., Orenstein, W. and Offit, P. (2003) *Vaccines*. Philidelphia: Saunders.

Porritt, J. (2005) 'Healthy environment–healthy people: the link between sustainable development and health', *Public Health*, 119: 952–3.

Power, C., Lake, J. K. and Cole, T. J. (1997) 'Measurement and long-term health risks of child and adolescent fatness', *International Journal of Obesity and Related Metabolic Disorders*, 21: 507–26.

Primary Care Group London Network for Nurses and Midwives (2007) *Commissioning a Patient-led NHS: A Toolkit for Nurses*. London: Primary Care Group London Network for Nurses and Midwives.

Pring, R. (2000) *Philosophy of Education Research*. New York: Continuum.

Public Health (Control of Disease) Act 1984 (1984). London: The Stationery Office.

Public Health Resource Unit (2007) *Public Health Workforce Framework*. Oxford: PHRU.

Public Health (Infectious Disease) regulation (1998). London: The Stationery Office.

Putnam, R. D. (1995) 'Bowling alone: America's declining social capital', *Journal of Democracy*, 6: 65–78.

Putnam, R. D. (2007) 'E pluribus unum: diversity and community in the twenty-first century: the 2006 Johan Skytte Prize Lecture', *Scandinavian Political Studies*, 30(2): 137–74.

Quarantelli, E. L. (ed.) (1998) *What is Disaster?* New York: Routledge.

Rains, J. C., Penzien, D. B. and Lipchik, G. L. (2006) 'Behavioural facilitation of medical treatment for headache – Part 2: theoretical models and behavioural strategies for improving adherence', *American Headache Society*, 46: 1395–403.

RCSLT (Royal College of Speech and Language Therapy) (n.d.) *Service Specification*. Retrieved 18 January 2008, from http://www.rcslt.org/resources/managers_resources/service_spec

Reed, J., Inglis, P., Cook, G., Clarke, C. and Cook, M. (2007) 'Specialist nurses for older people: implications from UK development sites', *Journal of Advanced Nursing*, 58(4): 368–76.

Reid, J., Jarvis, R., Richardson, J. and Stewart, A. G. (2005) *Responding to Chronic Environmental Problems in Cheshire and Merseyside – Systems and Procedures*. Retrieved 27 June 2007, from http://www.hpa.org.uk/chemicals/reports/CHAPR4_May2005.pdf

Replacement of treatability and care tests, Mental Health Act (2007).

Richards, H. L., Fortune, D. G. and Griffiths, C. E. M. (2005) 'Adherence to treatment in patients with psoriasis', *European Academy of Dermatology and Venereology*, 52: 468–73.

Richardson, L. and Le Grande, J. (2002) *Outsider and Insider Expertise: The Responses of Residents of Deprived Neighbourhoods to an Academic Definition of Social Exclusion*. London: London School of Economics, Centre for Analysis of Social Exclusion.

Rissel, C. (1994) 'Empowerment: The holy grail of health promotion', *Health Promotion International*, 9: 39–47.

Robinson, T. (2001) 'Television and childhood obesity', *Pediatric Clinics of North America*, 48(4): 1017–25.

Roche, M. (2004) 'Complicated problems, complicated solutions? Homelessness and joined up policy responses', *Social Policy and Administration*, 38(7): 758–74.

Roger, A. and Pilgrim, D. (2005) *A Sociology of Mental Health and Illness*, 3rd edn. Maidenhead: Open University Press.

Rogers, A. C. (1997) 'Vulnerability, health and healthcare', *Journal of Advanced Nursing*, 28: 65–72.

Rogers, B. (2003) *Occupational and Environmental Health: Concepts and Practice*. New York: Saunders.

Rogers, W. A. (2004) 'Ethical issues in public health: a qualitative study of public health practice in Scotland', *Journal of Epidemiology and Community Health*, 8: 446–50.

Rose, M. H. and Killien, M. (1983) 'Risk and vulnerability: a case for differentiation', *Advances in Nursing Science*, 5: 60–78.

Rowland, H. J. and Cooper, P. (1983) *Environment and Health*. London: Edward Arnold.

Runciman, P., Watson, H., McIntosh, J. and Tolson, D. (2006) 'Community nurses' health promotion work with older people', *Journal of Advanced Nursing*, 55(1): 46–57.

Ryan, J. M. Mahoney, P. F., Greaves, I. and Bowyer, G. (2002) *Conflict and Catastrophe Medicine: A Practical Guide*. London: Springer.

Rycroft-Malone, J. et al. (2004) ' What counts as evidence in evidence-based practice', *Journal of Advanced Nursing*, 47(1): 81–90.

Sackett, D. and Parkes, J. (1998) 'Teaching critical appraisal: no quick fixes', *Can Med Assoc J*, 158(2): 203–4.

Sackett, D. L., Rosenberg, W. M. C., Muir Gray, J. A., Haynes, R. B. and Richardson, W. S. (1996) 'Evidence based medicine: what it is and what it isn't', *British Medical Journal*, 312: 1085–6.

Sahota, P., Rudolph, M., Dixey, R., Hill, J. and Cade, J. (2001) 'Evaluation of implementation and effect of primary school based intervention to reduce risk factors for obesity', *British Medical Journal*, 323: 1027.

Salisbury, D., Beverley, P. and Miller, E. (2002) 'Vaccine programmes and policies', *British Medical Bulletin*, 62: 201–11.

Salisbury, D., Ramsay, M. and Noakes, K. (2006) *Immunisation Against Infectious Disease*. London: The Stationery Office.

Salmon, D. A. and Omer, S. B. (2006) 'Individual freedoms versus collective responsibility: immunization decision-making in the face of occasionally competing values online', *Emerging Themes in Epidemiology*, 3: 13.

Salmond, S. W. (2007) 'Advancing evidence based practice: a primer', *Orthopaedic Nursing*, 26(2): 114–23.

Saracci, R. (1999) 'Epidemiology in progress: thoughts, tensions and targets', *International Journal of Epidemiology*, 28(5): 997–9.

Scamber, G. (2004) *Medical Sociology: Major Themes in Health and Social Welfare*. London: Routledge.

Schama, S. (1995) *Landscape and Memory*. London: HarperCollins.

SCMH (2004) *Better Must Come. From Mental Health Services to Employment: Black Men Moving On*. London: The Sainsbury Centre for Mental Health.

SCMH (2007) *Policy Paper 8: Mental Health at Work: Developing the Business Case*. London: The Sainsbury Centre for Mental Health.

Scott, L. (2003) 'Vulnerability, need and significant harm: an analysis tool', *Community Practitioner*, 763: 468–73.

Scott-Samuel, A. (1998) 'Health impact assessment – theory into practice', *J Epidemiol Community Health*, 52: 704–5

Scott-Samuel, A., Birley, M. and Ardern, K. (2001) *The Merseyside Guidelines for Health Impact Assessment*, 3rd edn. London: International Health Impact Assessment Consortium.

Scriven, A. and Garmen, S. (2007) *Public Health: Social Context and Action*. London: McGraw-Hill.

Seale, C. (2003) *Media and Health*. London: Sage.

Seedhouse, D. (2006) *What Is Mental Health in Mental Health Promotion Across the Lifespan*. Milton Keynes: Open University Press.

Sellman, D. (2005) 'Towards an understanding of nursing as a response to human vulnerability', *Nursing Philosophy*, 6: 2–10.

Seo, D. C., Nehl, E., Agley, J. and Ma, S. M. (2007) 'Relations between physical activity and behavioural and perceptual correlates among midwestern college students', *J Am Coll Health*, 56(2): 187–97.

SEU (Social Exclusion Unit) (1998) *Rough Sleeping: A Report by the Social Exclusion Unit*. London: SEU.

Shaw, I. F., Greene, J. C. and Mark, M. M. (2006) *The Sage Handbook of Evaluation*. London: Sage.

Sheppard, M. and Woodcock, J. (1999) 'Needs as an operating concept: the case of social work with children and families', *Child and Family Social Work*, 4: 67–76.

Shinn, M. (2007) 'International homelessness: policy, socio-cultural, and individual perspectives', *Journal of Social Issues*, 63(3): 657–77.

Shipp, J. C., Vargas, L., Hughes, T., Fox, E. and Gonzales, D. (1999) 'A successful, cost-effective diabetes treatment program in a university county hospital', *Drug Benefit Trends*, 11(3): 56–66.

Simpson, J. A. and Weiner, E. S. C. (1989) *The Oxford Dictionary*, 2nd edn. Oxford: Clarendon Press.

Singleton, N., Bumpstead, R., O'Brien, M., Lee, A. and Meltzer, H. (2000) *Psychiatric Morbidity among Adults Living in Private Households*. London: Social Survey Division of the Office for National Statistics.

Skärsäter, I. (2006) 'Parents with first time major depression: perceptions of social support for themselves and their children', *Scandinavian Journal of Caring Science*, 20(3): 308–14.

Skinner, T. C. (2004) 'Psychological barriers. Adherence to treatment: a major obstacle to reaching goals in type 2 diabetes', *European Journal of Endocrinology*, 151(2): 13–17.

Smith, B. J., Tang, K. C. and Nutbeam, D. (2006) 'WHO Health Promotion Glossary: new terms', *Health Promotion International*, 21(4).

Social Exclusion Task Force (2006) *The Report on Reaching Out: An Action Plan on Social Exclusion*. London: Social Exclusion Unit.

Social Exclusion Unit (1999) *Teenage Pregnancy*. London: The Stationary Office.

Social Science Research Unit (2005) *Reaching out to Pregnant Teenagers and Teenage Parents: Innovative Practice from Sure Start Plus Pilot Programmes*. London: SSRU.

Solar, O. and Irwin, A. (2007) *Discussion Paper for the Commission on Social Determinants of Health – Draft April 2007*. Geneva: World Health Organization.

SouthAfrica.info. (2007) Doing business: economic review. Retrieved 13 February 2008, from www.southafricainfo/doing_business/economy/econorevview.htm

Stacey, R. (2002) *Strategic Management and Organisational Dynamics: The Challenge of Complexity*. London: Prentice-Hall.

Statham, D. (2000) 'Guest Editorial: Partnership between health and social care', *Health and Social Care in the Community*, 8(2): 87–9.

Stephens, T. (1998) 'Physical activity and mental health in the United States and Canada: evidence from four population surveys', *Preventive Medicine*, 17: 35–47.

Steptoe, A., Wardle, J., Cui, W., Bellisle, F., Zotti, A. M., Baranyai, R. and Sanderman, R. (2002) 'Trends in smoking, diet, physical exercise, and attitudes toward health in European university students from 13 countries, 1990–2000', *Preventive Medicine*, 35(2): 97–104.

Stewart, A. G., Wilkinson, E. and Howard, C. (2005) '*Health:* a necessity for sustainable development'. Paper presented at the the World Summit on Sustainable Development.

Stock, C., Kücük, N., Miseviciene, I., Guillen-Grima, F., Petkeviciene, J. and Aguinaga-Ontoso, I. (2003) 'Differences in health complaints among university students from three European countries', *Preventive Medicine*, 37(6): 535–43.

Susser, M. (1999) 'Should the epidemiologist be a social scientist or a molecular biologist?' *International Journal of Epidemiology*, 28(5): 1019–22.

Susser, M. and Susser, E. (1996a) 'Choosing a future for epidemiology: 1. Eras and paradigms', *American Journal of Public Health*, 86(5): 668–73.

Susser, M. and Susser, E. (1996b) 'Choosing a future for epidemiology: 2 From black box to Chinese boxes and eco-epidemiology', *American Journal of Public Health*, 86(5): 674–7.

Swanson, D., Pintér, L., Bregha, F., Volkery, A. and Jacob, K. (2004) *National Strategies for Sustainable Development: Challenges, Approaches and Innovations in Strategic and Co-ordinated Action, Based on a 19-country Analysis*. Retrieved 13 February 2008, from http://www.iisd.org/pdf/2004/measure_nat_strategies_sd.pdf

Taylor, A. H., Doust, J. and Webborn, A. D. J. (1998) 'Randomised controlled trial to examine the effects of a GP exercise referral programme in Hailsham, East Sussex, on modifiable coronary heart disease risk factors', *Journal of Epidemiology and Community Health*, 52: 595–601.

Taylor, G., Easter, K. and Hegney, R. (2004) *Enhancing Occupational Safety and Health*. Burlington, MA: Elsevier Butterworth-Heinemann.

Taylor, L., Taske, N., Swann, C. and Waller, S. (2007) *Public Health Interventions to Promote Positive Mental Health and Prevent Mental Health Disorders among Adults. Evidence Briefing, National Institute for Clinical Excellence*. London: NICE.

Terry, L. L. (1964) 'The complex world of modern public health: the third annual Bronfman lecture', *Am J Public Health Nations Health*, 54(2): 189–95.

Themesl-Hubber, M., Hubbard, G. and Munro, P. (2007) 'Frail older people's experiences and use of health and social care services', *Journal of Advanced Nursing*, 15: 222–9.

Thomas, M. and Hynes, C. (1998) 'Acquiring knowledge', in T. Harrison (ed.), *Children and Sexuality – Perspectives in Healthcare*. London: Baillière, Tindall.

Thorogood, N. (1992) 'What is the relevance of sociology for health promotion?' in R. and M. G. Bunton (eds), *Health Promotion: Disciplines and Diversity*. London: Routledge.

Tones, K. and Green, J. (2004) *Health Promotion. Planning and Strategies*. London: Sage.

Tones, K. and Tilford, S. (2001) *Health Promotion Effectiveness, Efficiency and Equity*. Cheltenham: Nelson Thornes.

Townsend, P., Davidson, N. and Whithead, M. (1992) *The Black Report and the Health Divide: Inequalities in Health*. London: Penguin.

Travers, K. D. (1996) 'The social organization of nutritional inequities', *Social Science and Medicine*, 43: 543–53.

Trinder, L. and Reynolds, S. (2000) *Evidence-Based Practice. A Critical Appraisal*. Oxford: Blackwell Science.

Turner, B. S. (1991) 'Recent developments in the theory of the body', in M. Featherstone, M. Hepworth and B.S.Turner (eds), *The Body: Social Processes and Cultural Theory*. London: Sage.

The UK Law Statute Database, The Ministry of Justice (1985).

UK National Screening Committee (2003) *Criteria for Appraising the Viability, Effectiveness and Appropriatness of a Screening Programme*. Retrieved 12 December 2007, from http://www.library.nhs.uk/screening/

UK Public Health Association (2007) *Climates and Change – The Urgent Need to Connect Health and Sustainable Development*. London: UKPHA.

UNAIDS and World Health Organization (2004) *AIDS Epidemic Update. UNAIDS/04*. Geneva: UNAIDS and World Health Organization.

United Nations (1992) *'Agenda 21'*, in *Report of the United Nations*. Rio de Janeiro: United Nations.

United Nations (1997) *Programme for the Further Implementation of Agenda 21*. New York: United Nations.

United Nations (2002) *World Summit on Sustainable Development*. Johannesburg: United Nations.

University of Toronto (2007) *Health Promotion Programme Planning*. Toronto: University of Toronto.

US Census Bureau (2004) *International Population Reports WP/02*. Washington, DC: US Government Printing Office.

Vermeire, E., Hearnshaw, H., Van Royen, P. and Denekens, J. (2001) 'Patient adherence to treatment: three decades of research. A comprehensive review', *Journal of Clinical Pharmacy and Therapeutics*, 262: 331–4.

von Bertalanffy, L. (1968) *General Systems Theory*. New York: Brazilli.

von Schirnding, Y. (2002) *Health in Sustainable Development Planning: The Role of Indicators*. Retrieved 13 February 2008, from http://www.who.int/mediacentre/events/IndicatorsFrontpages.pdf

Vrijheid, M. (2000) 'Health effects of residence near hazardous waste landfill sites: a review of epidemiologic literature', *Environmental Health Perspectives*, 108(1): 101–12.

Wade, E., Smith, J., Peck, E. and Freeman, T. (2006) *Commissioning in the Reformed NHS: Policy into Practice*. Birmingham: University of Birmingham, Health Services Management Centre NHS Alliance.

Wagstaff, A. (2002) 'Poverty and health sector inequalities', *Bulletin of the World Health Organisation*, 80(2): 97–105.

Wakefield, A. J. et al. (1998) 'Ileal-lymphoid-nodular hyperplasia, non-specific colitis, and pervasive developmental disorder in children', *Lancet*, 351: 637–41

Waldron, I. (1980) 'Employment and women's health: An analysis of causal relationships', *International Journal of Health Services*, 10(3): 435–54.

Wankel, L. M. (1993) 'The importance of enjoyment to adherence and psychological benefits from physical activity', *International Journal of Sports Psychology*, 24: 151–69.

Wardle, J., Griffiths, J., Johnson, F. and Rapoport, L. (2000) 'Intentional weight control and food choice habits in a national representative sample of adults in the UK', *International Journal of Obesity and Related Metabolic Disorders*, 24: 534–40.

Wardle, J., Parmenter, K. and Waller, J. (2000) 'Nutrition knowledge and food intake', *Appetite*, 34: 269–75.

Wardle, J., Steptoe, A., Gulis, G., Sek, H., Todorova, I., Vogele, C. et al. (2004) 'Depression, perceived control, and life satisfaction in university students from central-Eastern and western Europe', *International Journal of Behavioural Medicine*, 11(1): 2–36.

Watterson, A. (2003) *Public Health Practice*. Basingstoke: Macmillan.

Weale, A. (2006) 'What is so good about citizens' involvement in healthcare?' in E. Andersson, J. Tritter and R. Wilson (eds), *Healthy Democracy*. London: Involve/ NCI.

Weed, D. (2002) 'Theory and practice in epidemiology', *Annals of the New York Academy of Sciences*, 954(1): 52–62.

Weinreich, P. and Saunderson, W. (2003) *Analysing Identity: Cross-Cultural, Societal and Clinical Contexts*. London: Routledge.

Weiss, N. S., Anderson, R. M. and Lasker, R. D. (2002) 'Making the most of collaboration: exploring the relationship between partnership synergy and partnership functioning', *Health Educ Behav*, 29: 683–98.

Welsh Assembly Government (2006) *Chief Medical Officer's Report Series Wales 2: Health in Local Areas: A Compendium of Maps*. Retrieved 20 August 2007, from http://new.wales.gov.uk/topics/health/ocmo/communications/reports/maps?lang=en

Wenzal, E. (1997) 'A comment on health promotion settings', *Journal of Health Promotion*, 1: 1–19.

Wheway, R. and Millward, A. (1997) *Child's Play: Facilitating Play on Housing Estates*. London: Chartered Institute of Housing.

Whitehead, D. (2000) 'Using mass media within health-promoting practice: a nursing perspective', *Journal of Advanced Nursing*, 32(4): 80 7–16.

Whitehead, D. (2003) 'Health promotion and health education viewed as symbiotic paradigms: bridging the gap between them', *Journal of Clinical Nursing*, 12: 796–805.

Whitehead, E. (2001) 'Teenage pregnancy: on the road to social death', *International Journal of Nursing Studies*, 38: 437–46.

Whitehead, M. (ed.) (1995) *Tackling Inequalities: A Review of Policy Initiatives.* London: King's Fund.

WHO (World Health Organization) (1948) *Constitution of the World Health Organization.* Geneva: WHO.

WHO (1978) *The Alma Ata Declaration.* Geneva: WHO.

WHO (1984) *Health for All Targets.* Copenhagen: WHO.

WHO (1985) *Targets for Health For All.* Copenhagen: Regional Office for Europe.

WHO (1986) *Ottawa Charter for Health Promotion.* Geneva: WHO.

WHO (1993) *The Health of Young People, A Challenge and a Promise.* Geneva: WHO.

WHO (1997) *The Jakata Declaration on Health Promotion Offers a Vision and Focus for Health Promotion into the Next Century.* Geneva: WHO.

WHO (1998) 'Resolution of the Executive Board of the WHO on health promotion', *Health Promotion International*, 13(266).

WHO (2004) *Guiding Principle for Feeding Infants and Young Children During Emergencies.* Geneva: WHO.

WHO (2005d) *Effective Media Communication During Public Health Emergencies.* Geneva: WHO.

WHO (1998) *Health Promotion Glossary.* Geneva: WHO.

WHO (1999) 'Health impact assessment: main concepts and suggested approach: Gothenburg Consensus Papere'. Paper presented at the WHO Regional Office for Europe.

WHO (2000) *Smallpox (HTML).* Geneva: WHO.

WHO (2002) *Environmental Health Criteria for Fluorides.* Geneva: WHO.

WHO (2003) *Social Determinants of Health: The Solid Facts.* Geneva: WHO.

WHO (2004) *Active Ageing: Towards Age Friendly Primary Healthcare.* Retrieved 10 November 2007, from http://whqlibdoc.who.int/publications/2004/9241592184. pdf

WHO (2005) *Sustainable Development and Healthy Environments Highlights 2004: Protecting Human Health through Scientific Evidence, Reasonable Caution and Strategic Partnerships.* Geneva: WHO.

WHO (2007) *Global Strategy on Diet, Physical Activity and Health: Obesity and Overweight.* Geneva: WHO.

WHO (n.d.) *World Summit on Sustainable Development.* Retrieved 13 February 2008, from http://www.who.int/wssd/en/

Wilcox, D. (1994) *Effective Participation.* London: Partnership Books.

Williams, R. (1998) *Keywords: A Vocabulary of Culture and Society, Revised and Expanded.* London: Fontana.

Wilkinson, R. and Marmot, M. (2003) *Social Determinants of Health. The Solid Facts.* Geneva: WHO.

Wills, J. and Earle, S. (2007) 'Theoretical perspectives on promoting public health', in S. Earle, E. C. Lloyd, M. Sidell and S. Spurr (eds), *Theory and Research in Promoting Public Health.* London: Sage in association with Open University.

Wilson, E. O. (1984) *Biophilia: The Human Bond with Other Species*. Cambridge, MA: Harvard University Press.

Wilson, J. M. G. and Jungner, G. (1968) *Principles and Practice of Screening for Disease*. Geneva: WHO.

Wood-Harper, J. (2005) 'Informing education policy on MMR: Balancing individual freedom and collective responsibilities for the promotion of public health', *Nursing Ethics*, 12: 43–58.

Woodin, J. (2006) 'Healthcare commissioning and contracting', in K. Walshe and J. Smith (eds), *Healthcare Management*. Maidenhead: Open University Press.

Woodroffe, C., Glickmanm, M., Barker, M. and Power, C. (1993) *Children, Teenagers and Health: The key data*. Buckingham: Open University Press.

World Bank (1993) *World Development Report 1993: Investing in Health*. New York: Oxford University Press.

World Commission on Environment and Development (WCED) (1987) *Our Common Future*. Switzerland: United Nations.

Wright, J. (1998) *Health Needs Assessment in Practice*. London: BMJ Books.

Wright Foundation Conference (2003) *4th National GP Referral*. Birmingham.

Wynn, T. A., Johnson, R. E., Fouad, M., Holt, C., Scarinci, I., Nagy, C. et al. (2006) 'Addressing disparities through coalition building: Alabama REACH 2010 lessons learning', *J Healthcare Poor Underserved*, 17(2): 55–77.

Young, I. and Whitehead, M. (1993) 'Back to the future: our social history and its impact on health education', *Health Education Journal*, 52(3): 114–19.

Zakocs, R. C. and Edwards, E. M. (2006) 'What explains community coalition effectiveness? A review of the literature', *American Journal of Preventive Medicine*, 30(4): 351–336.

Zubin and Spring (1977) 'Vulnerability: a new view of schizophrenia', *Journal of Abnormal Psychology*, 86: 260–66.

key concepts
in public health

Index

index

index

Foucault, 32, 34
fourth era, 22

gender, 32, 89–90, 160, 198, 204, 259
General Medical Council, 53
general practitioner, 53, 166, 250
geographical areas, 26, 28, 90, 96
germ theory/era, 7, 22–3
globalisation, 31,178,
global tobacco control, 12
global warming, 175, 253
Goffman, Irving, 98–101
governance, 76, 190, 265
government intervention, 255
green exercise, gym, space, 164–7

hard to reach groups, 84, 214, 222, 239
health beliefs, 33, 243, 253, 263
health education, 32, 33, 95, 146, 149,
    159, 215, 222, 243, 268
health equity audit, 28
health field concept, 16, 147
health gap, widening, 26–8
health impact assessment, 19, 130–4, 146
health improvement initiatives, 12, 13
health inequalities, 11, 18, 26, 74, 92,
    120, 133, 159, 212, 237, 265, 270
health literacy, 78–83, 183
health needs assessment, 113–18, 234,
    238, 274, 276
health outcomes, 14, 26–8, 160, 208, 238
health policies, 48, 90, 146, 202, 236
health promoting schools, 123
health promotion, 145–51, 159, 198,
    207, 210, 225
health protection, 135–40
Health Protection Agency, 9, 10, 46,
    140, 168
health protection response, 172
health and safety executive,
    50, 136, 272–4
health visitor, 8, 24, 57, 59, 116, 237, 238
health and wellbeing, 93, 104, 118,
    146, 164–7, 203–7, 241–5, 262
healthy schools, 242–4
Healthwise project, 203–6
heart disease, 8, 19, 27, 34, 47, 114,
    166, 208–12, 254, 257
hepatitis B, 70–2, 141–2
herd immunity, 141, 142, 253

Hib vaccine, 143–4
hierarchy of evidence, 194–6
HIV/AIDS, 186, 187, 199
home visiting, intensive, 237–8
homeless, 104, 214, 249
homelessness, 107–8, 200, 266–9
horizon scanning, 122
hospital based services, 23
human rights, 13, 32, 50, 74,
    96, 254, 268
Human Rights Act, 54, 227

illegal substances, 243, 247
illiteracy, 79, 81, 189
immune response, 140, 142
immune system, 140, 144, 160
immunisation, 22, 52, 72, 140–5, 198
    childhood programme, 143
immunity, 140–4
impetigo, 24
incidence of disease, 85, 115, 141–2
incidence and prevalence, 37, 171
industrial revolution, 5
industrialisation, 31, 77
inequalities in health, 20, 23, 25–30,
    96, 197, 264
infant mortality, 7, 43
infectious diseases, 8, 9, 23, 51,
    135–7, 140–2
influence intergenerational, 75, 237
influenza, 141–2, 177, 275
interdisciplinary, 24–5, 189, 199
internal market, 219
internet, 83–4, 182
isolation, 27, 53, 101, 167, 264

Japanese encephalitis, 142
joined up approaches, 14, 27, 228
joint working, 88, 187, 233

King's Fund, 59, 254
Koch, Robert, 7

Lalonde Report, 16, 147
lay health beliefs, 33
leadership, 55–61, 188–90, 221–2, 256
leadership awareness model, 56, 59, 60
leadership at the point of care, 59, 291
Leading Empowered Organisations
    (LEO), 59

index

key concepts
in public health

Research Methods Books
from SAGE

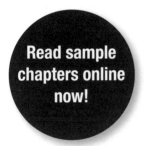
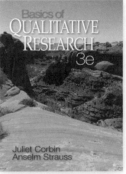

Basics of
QUALITATIVE
RESEARCH
3e

Juliet Corbin
Anselm Strauss

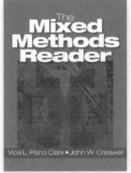

The
Mixed
Methods
Reader

Vicki L. Plano Clark ▪ John W. Creswell

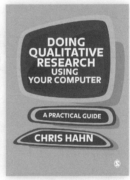

DOING
QUALITATIVE
RESEARCH
USING
YOUR COMPUTER

A PRACTICAL GUIDE

CHRIS HAHN

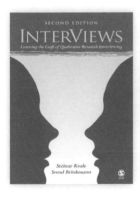

SECOND EDITION
INTERVIEWS
Learning the Craft of Qualitative Research Interviewing

Steinar Kvale
Svend Brinkmann

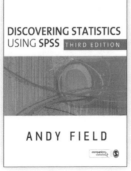

DISCOVERING STATISTICS
USING SPSS THIRD EDITION

ANDY FIELD

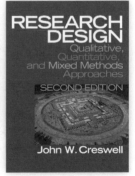

RESEARCH
DESIGN
Qualitative,
Quantitative,
and Mixed Methods
Approaches

SECOND EDITION

John W. Creswell

www.sagepub.co.uk

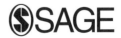

The Qualitative Research Kit

Edited by Uwe Flick

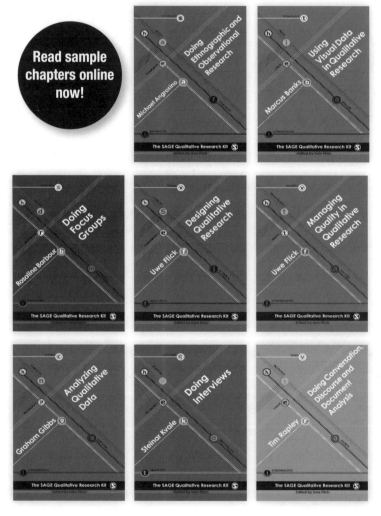

Read sample chapters online now!

Doing Ethnographic and Observational Research — Michael Angrosino

Using Visual Data in Qualitative Research — Marcus Banks

Doing Focus Groups — Rosaline Barbour

Designing Qualitative Research — Uwe Flick

Managing Quality in Qualitative Research — Uwe Flick

Analyzing Qualitative Data — Graham Gibbs

Doing Interviews — Steinar Kvale

Doing Conversation, Discourse and Document Analysis — Tim Rapley

www.sagepub.co.uk

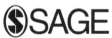